Home Apothecary For Beginners

600+ Forgotten Herbal Remedies for Health and Wellness!

Barbara Nicole

Published by Barbara Nicole

First Edition, 2024

CONTENTS

A QUICK FAVOR BEFORE YOU BEGIN

Hi there! Before you dive into this book, I wanted to ask for a small favor. If you find this guide helpful, inspiring, or even just a little fun, would you consider leaving a quick review on Amazon? Your feedback not only means the world to me, but it also helps other curious readers discover this book and start their own herbal journey.

It doesn't have to be long—just a few words about what you loved (or even what could be better!) makes a huge difference. Think of it as a way to pass the gift of herbal wisdom along to others. Thank you for your support—it truly keeps this dream alive!

With gratitude,
Barbara Nicole

WELCOME TO YOUR HOME APOTHECARY

Imagine standing in your kitchen, surrounded by jars filled with fragrant herbs, colorful flowers, and dried roots. A kettle of water simmers gently on the stove, waiting to steep your latest herbal creation. On your shelves sit tinctures, teas, and salves you've crafted yourself, each ready to ease a headache, soothe a sore throat, or simply bring calm after a long day. This is the magic of having your own home apothecary—a place where nature meets wellness, and you take an active role in your health and that of your family.

Welcome, friend, to your journey into herbal healing.

This book isn't just a guide; it's your companion. Together, we'll explore the timeless wisdom of herbal remedies, empowering you to create a home apothecary that's as simple or as robust as you'd like. Whether you're completely new to herbal medicine or have already dabbled with a few teas and tinctures, this book will meet you where you are, helping you build confidence and knowledge step by step.

Why Start a Home Apothecary?

For centuries, before the rise of modern medicine, families relied on home apothecaries to care for their health. These spaces were stocked with dried herbs, homemade salves, and other natural remedies, often passed down through generations. A home apothecary wasn't just about treating illness; it was about cultivating a lifestyle rooted in self-reliance, nature, and care.

Today, many of us are rediscovering the beauty of these simple, natural practices. A home apothecary allows you to:

- **Take control of your health**: Knowing how to use herbs empowers you to address common ailments naturally and effectively.
- **Live more sustainably**: By growing, foraging, or sourcing your own herbs, you can reduce your reliance on mass-produced, chemical-laden products.
- **Reconnect with nature**: Working with herbs invites us to slow down and appreciate the healing power of the earth.
- **Nurture your loved ones**: There's something deeply satisfying about offering a remedy you've created with your own hands.

What You'll Find in This Book

This book is designed to guide you on your herbal journey from the ground up, making the process approachable and enjoyable. You'll learn how to:

- Build a home apothecary with must-have herbs, tools, and ingredients.
- Create simple yet effective remedies like teas, tinctures, salves, and tonics.
- Address common ailments like colds, headaches, and digestive troubles using natural solutions.
- Embrace herbs as part of your daily life, for everything from skincare to emotional wellness.
- Grow your herbal knowledge, whether through gardening, foraging, or advanced techniques.

Throughout the book, you'll find clear instructions, practical recipes, and plenty of encouragement. I've included personal anecdotes, tips, and troubleshooting advice to help you feel supported every step of the way.

A Personal Note: My Journey into Herbalism

My journey into herbalism began during a time of overwhelm. Like so many others, I felt increasingly disconnected from the natural world, spending my days glued to screens and relying on store-bought products for every little need. A persistent bout of stress and insomnia finally led me to look for alternatives.

One evening, I stumbled upon a simple chamomile tea recipe for sleep. I made it with no great expectations, but something about the ritual—boiling water, steeping the delicate flowers, and sipping that warm, soothing brew—stayed with me. I slept better that night, but more importantly, I felt a spark of curiosity. What else could herbs do?

That spark led me to dive deeper into the world of herbalism. I started small, experimenting with basic remedies and reading every book I could find. Slowly, I began building my home apothecary—a few jars on the counter became shelves stocked with vibrant herbs and homemade creations. Today, herbs are part of my daily life, and I can't imagine living without them.

Herbalism has taught me that healing is a process, not just for the body but for the soul. It's about learning to care for ourselves and others in ways that are thoughtful, intentional, and connected to the natural rhythms of life.

How to Begin

Starting your own home apothecary doesn't have to be complicated. In fact, it's best to begin simply. Start with just a handful of versatile herbs, like chamomile for calming teas, peppermint for digestive support, or calendula for skin healing. Learn to prepare these in basic ways—teas, tinctures, or salves—and grow your knowledge gradually.

As you explore this book, you'll find that herbal medicine is as much about the journey as it is about the remedies. With each recipe you try, each herb you learn to work with, you'll deepen your relationship with nature and your understanding of your own body.

A Few Words on Herbal Safety

Herbs are powerful allies, but like anything, they should be used thoughtfully. Throughout this book, you'll find guidance on dosage, preparation, and safety to ensure your remedies are as effective and gentle as possible.

It's important to remember: herbal remedies are not a replacement for professional medical care when it's needed. Always consult with a healthcare provider for serious or ongoing health concerns, and take time to educate yourself about the herbs you're using.

Let's Begin!

Your home apothecary is more than a collection of jars and remedies. It's a reflection of your commitment to a natural, intentional way of living. As you take this first step, know that you're reconnecting with ancient traditions and empowering yourself to care for your health and the health of those you love.

So grab a cup of tea (maybe chamomile or peppermint!) and settle in. Let's build your home apothecary together, one herb, one remedy, and one discovery at a time.

Welcome to the world of herbal healing—I'm so glad you're here.

THE HEALING POWER OF HERBAL REMEDIES

Throughout history, humans have turned to plants for healing, nourishment, and vitality. Long before the advent of modern medicine, herbal remedies were the foundation of health and wellness, connecting us to the natural world in deeply profound ways. Even now, in an era of cutting-edge pharmaceuticals and advanced medical technology, herbs remain a gentle yet powerful way to support the body's natural ability to heal.

This chapter is all about helping you rediscover the healing power of herbal remedies—what makes them effective, how they work in harmony with the body, and why they've stood the test of time. My hope is that you'll see herbs not just as tools for treating illness, but as allies in creating a life of balance and well-being.

Why Herbs Are So Powerful

Herbs work in harmony with the body rather than against it. Unlike synthetic drugs, which often target a single symptom or system, herbs are full of complex compounds that address multiple aspects of health simultaneously. For example:

- **Peppermint** not only soothes indigestion but also helps relieve headaches and clear sinus congestion.
- **Chamomile** calms an anxious mind, supports restful sleep, and eases inflammation in the digestive system.

- **Turmeric** acts as a potent anti-inflammatory, helps manage pain, and supports liver detoxification.

What makes herbs unique is their **holistic approach to healing**. Instead of suppressing symptoms, they work to restore balance in the body, addressing root causes while supporting the body's natural healing mechanisms.

How Herbal Remedies Work

Plants contain a variety of bioactive compounds—such as alkaloids, tannins, flavonoids, and volatile oils—that work together to support health. Let's break it down a little further:

1. **Adaptogens: Restoring Balance**
   Some herbs, like ashwagandha, holy basil, and ginseng, are known as **adaptogens**. These herbs help the body adapt to stress, whether physical, mental, or emotional. They regulate cortisol levels, strengthen the adrenal glands, and improve resilience over time.

2. **Anti-Inflammatories: Reducing Pain and Swelling**
   Chronic inflammation is at the root of many modern health issues, from arthritis to cardiovascular disease. Herbs like turmeric, ginger, and calendula work to calm inflammation and reduce pain naturally.

3. **Antimicrobials: Fighting Infections**
   Herbs like garlic, thyme, and oregano are natural antibiotics and antivirals, helping the body fight off bacterial, viral, and fungal infections without disrupting the gut microbiome like synthetic antibiotics often do.

4. **Nervines: Calming the Nervous System**
   Stress and anxiety are common struggles today, and herbal nervines—such as valerian, lemon balm, and passionflower —can gently calm an overactive nervous system without the

side effects of prescription medications.

5. **Digestive Tonics: Supporting Gut Health**
   From peppermint to fennel, many herbs act as digestive aids, easing bloating, nausea, and indigestion. Others, like licorice root and slippery elm, help heal and protect the lining of the stomach and intestines.

The Ancient Roots of Herbal Healing

Herbal remedies have been used in nearly every culture and tradition, often passed down through oral history or sacred texts.

- **Traditional Chinese Medicine (TCM):** In TCM, herbs are used alongside acupuncture and dietary therapy to balance the body's energy, or Qi. Ingredients like ginseng, astragalus, and ginger are staples of this centuries-old practice.
- **Ayurveda:** The ancient Indian system of medicine views herbs as tools to balance the doshas (vata, pitta, and kapha). Tulsi (holy basil), turmeric, and triphala are commonly used to bring harmony to mind and body.
- **European Herbalism:** The herbal traditions of Europe, particularly those of the Celts, Greeks, and Romans, have been preserved for thousands of years. Chamomile, lavender, and yarrow are just a few of the herbs central to these practices.
- **Indigenous Traditions:** Many Indigenous cultures around the world, from North America to Africa, have rich herbal traditions, using plants for physical, emotional, and spiritual healing. Sage, echinacea, and cedar are widely respected for their medicinal and ceremonial uses.

The Benefits of Herbal Remedies Today

Herbal medicine remains just as relevant today as it was in ancient times. In fact, many modern pharmaceuticals are derived from the same plant compounds herbalists have used for generations. For example:

- **Aspirin** was inspired by salicylic acid, a compound found in willow bark.
- **Digoxin**, used for heart conditions, comes from foxglove.
- **Quinine**, a treatment for malaria, is derived from the bark of the cinchona tree.

But unlike isolated pharmaceutical compounds, herbs offer a **synergy** of active constituents, which often makes them more effective with fewer side effects.

Beyond treating illness, herbs also offer support for daily wellness. For instance:

- A cup of **peppermint tea** can energize you without the jitters of caffeine.
- A daily dose of **elderberry syrup** can strengthen your immune system and keep colds at bay.
- A lavender-infused bath can relax your muscles and calm your mind.

Herbs as a Way of Life

Herbal remedies aren't just about treating symptoms—they're about adopting a lifestyle of mindful, proactive care. When you integrate herbs into your daily routine, you naturally become more attuned to your body's needs and rhythms.

For example:

- Drinking a calming **lemon balm tea** after a long day can signal to your body that it's time to unwind.
- Adding fresh **parsley or cilantro** to your meals offers a natural dose of antioxidants and detoxifying compounds.
- Applying a simple **calendula salve** to a cut or scrape reminds you of the power of gentle, natural healing.

Over time, these small choices add up to create a life that feels more connected—to nature, to your body, and to the wisdom of those who came before us.

The Gift of Connection

One of the most beautiful aspects of working with herbs is how it deepens your connection to the natural world. You begin to notice the plants growing around you, their shapes and scents, their unique personalities. The changing seasons take on new meaning as you forage wild herbs in spring, harvest flowers in summer, and gather roots in autumn.

This connection goes beyond physical healing—it's emotional and spiritual, too. Herbalism invites us to slow down, to listen, and to appreciate the gifts that the earth offers us.

Let's Rediscover What's Been Forgotten

In many ways, herbalism is about remembering—remembering the remedies our ancestors used, the plants that grow in our own backyards, and the profound connection we have to the natural world. It's about reclaiming the knowledge that's been forgotten, dusting it off, and making it a vibrant part of our modern lives.

Whether you're easing a cough with thyme tea, calming your mind with lavender, or tending a tiny herb garden on your windowsill, you're joining a tradition that stretches back thousands of years.

So, let's get started. Together, we'll learn how to harness the healing power of herbs in ways that are simple, practical, and transformative. Your journey into herbal healing begins here, and I'm honored to walk this path with you.

HOW TO USE THIS BOOK: A QUICK GUIDE

Whether you're a complete beginner or someone who's experimented with herbal teas and remedies before, this book is designed to meet you where you are. The chapters ahead will take you step by step through the process of creating herbal remedies, understanding how herbs work, and incorporating them into your daily life. But this isn't just a book to read—it's a resource to explore, experiment with, and return to whenever you need inspiration or guidance.

Here's how to get the most out of it:

---

1. Start Where You Are

This book is designed for all levels of experience. If you're brand new to herbalism, you'll find detailed explanations of the basics —what tools you need, how to prepare remedies, and which herbs are the most versatile for beginners.

If you already have some knowledge of herbs, feel free to jump straight into the recipes, remedy ideas, or more advanced sections, like combining herbs for maximum effectiveness or growing your own herb garden. There's no "wrong" way to use this book—make it your own!

---

2. Explore at Your Own Pace

This book isn't meant to be read cover to cover in one sitting.

Think of it as your personal herbal companion, here to support you as you build confidence in working with herbs.

- **Are you dealing with a specific issue?** Jump to Part 2, "Remedies for Everyday Ailments," and find targeted solutions for colds, headaches, digestive troubles, or other common concerns.
- **Curious about beauty and self-care?** Head to Part 3, where you'll find herbal recipes for glowing skin, strong hair, and more.
- **Looking for ways to relax or improve sleep?** Check out Part 4, which is all about emotional and mental wellness.

No matter what chapter you land on, you'll find actionable tips and clear instructions to help you incorporate herbal healing into your life.

---

3. Learn by Doing

The best way to learn herbalism is to get hands-on! This book is packed with recipes, remedies, and preparation techniques that you can try right away. Each recipe is written with beginners in mind, with simple, step-by-step instructions.

Here's how you can get started:

- **Follow the "Simple Preparations" section in Part 1** to learn the basics of making teas, tinctures, salves, and more.
- Gather just a few herbs to begin with (we'll go over the must-haves for a beginner's apothecary) and experiment with the recipes that call to you.
- Keep a notebook or herbal log to track your progress—write down what you try, how it works, and how it makes you feel. You'll find a DIY Herbal Log Template in the appendices to

help you get started.

The more you practice, the more confident you'll become. Remember, herbalism is as much about the journey as the destination.

---

4. Use the Quick Reference Tools

I've included some handy tools to help you quickly find what you need:

- **Symptom-to-Remedy Finder (Appendix):** This is your shortcut for matching common ailments (like a sore throat or headache) with effective herbal remedies.
- **Herbal Quick Reference Guide (Appendix):** A one-stop resource for learning about individual herbs, their properties, and how to use them.
- **DIY Herbal Log Template (Appendix):** A simple way to keep track of your experiments and results as you grow your skills.

Bookmark these sections so you can easily flip to them whenever you need a refresher.

---

5. Focus on Herbal Safety

Your health and safety are my top priorities. Throughout this book, you'll find clear instructions for proper dosages, safety tips, and precautions for each herb and recipe.

Here are some general guidelines to keep in mind as you dive in:

- **Start slow:** Begin with mild herbs and small amounts until you understand how your body responds.
- **Know your herbs:** Some herbs aren't suitable for children,

pregnant or nursing women, or people with certain health conditions. I've included safety notes wherever applicable, but always do additional research if you have specific concerns.

- **When in doubt, consult a professional:** Herbal remedies are a wonderful complement to professional healthcare, but they're not a replacement. For serious or ongoing health issues, always consult with a qualified healthcare provider.

As long as you approach herbalism with care and respect, you'll be able to enjoy its benefits safely and effectively.

---

6. Personalize Your Herbal Journey

One of the most rewarding parts of herbalism is that it's deeply personal. Every body is unique, and what works for one person might not work for another. That's why I encourage you to customize the recipes and remedies in this book to suit your own needs.

- **Experiment with flavors:** If you find a tea blend too strong, try adjusting the ratios or adding a touch of honey.
- **Try different herbs:** Don't have chamomile on hand? Substitute it with lemon balm or lavender.
- **Tailor remedies to your lifestyle:** Busy schedule? Focus on quick, easy remedies like herbal teas and tinctures that take just minutes to prepare.

Herbalism is as much an art as it is a science. Over time, you'll develop your own style and preferences—and that's part of the fun!

---

7. Embrace the Seasons

Herbs have a beautiful way of helping us connect with the

natural rhythms of the earth. This book includes seasonal suggestions to help you align your remedies with the changing cycles of nature:

- **In spring**, explore cleansing and rejuvenating herbs like dandelion and nettle.
- **In summer**, focus on cooling herbs like mint and hibiscus to beat the heat.
- **In autumn**, support your immune system with elderberry and echinacea.
- **In winter**, turn to warming herbs like ginger and cinnamon for comfort and resilience.

Let the seasons guide your herbal practice, and you'll find even more joy in your remedies.

---

8. Stay Curious and Keep Learning

Herbalism is an ancient practice with infinite depth. This book is just the beginning of your journey! As you grow more confident, you may want to explore advanced techniques, like making your own herbal syrups or foraging wild plants.

To help you continue learning, I've included a list of recommended resources in the appendices, including books, websites, and online courses. I also encourage you to connect with local herbalists, join an herbal study group, or take a workshop—it's a wonderful way to deepen your knowledge and meet like-minded people.

HERBAL SAFETY: DOSAGE, PRECAUTIONS, AND BEST PRACTICES

Herbs are nature's medicine, offering gentle and effective ways to support health and wellness. However, it's important to remember that "natural" doesn't always mean "safe." Just like pharmaceuticals, herbs contain powerful active compounds that require thoughtful use. Proper dosage, awareness of potential side effects, and understanding how to handle herbs safely are essential steps in your herbal journey. This chapter will guide you through the foundational principles of herbal safety so you can approach remedies with confidence and care.

---

1. Respect the Power of Herbs

Although herbs are often milder than synthetic drugs, they still interact with your body in significant ways. Inappropriate dosages, improper preparation, or using an herb without understanding its properties can lead to unwanted side effects or complications. For example:

- **Chamomile**, a calming herb, can trigger allergic reactions in people sensitive to ragweed.
- **St. John's Wort**, an excellent herb for mild depression, can interact dangerously with certain medications like

antidepressants and birth control pills.

- **Licorice Root**, while soothing to the digestive system, can raise blood pressure if consumed in large amounts.

The key to safe herbal practice is to educate yourself about the herbs you're using and to always start small, paying close attention to how your body responds.

---

2. Start with a Patch Test

If you're using a topical remedy—such as a salve or oil—always perform a patch test before applying it to a larger area of skin.

How to do a patch test:

1. Apply a small amount of the remedy to the inside of your wrist or elbow.
2. Wait 24 hours to see if there's any redness, itching, swelling, or irritation.
3. If your skin reacts negatively, avoid using that herb topically.

This simple step is especially important for people with sensitive skin or known allergies.

---

3. Understand Proper Dosage

Herbs are not a "one-size-fits-all" solution. Dosage depends on factors like your age, weight, health condition, and sensitivity to herbs.

General Dosage Guidelines

- **Teas:** 1–2 teaspoons of dried herbs per 8 ounces of water, steeped for 5–15 minutes. Drink 1–3 cups daily.

- **Tinctures:** 20–40 drops (1–2 droppers full), 1–3 times a day, diluted in water or tea.
- **Capsules or Powders:** Follow the manufacturer's instructions, as concentrations can vary widely.

It's always better to start with the lowest effective dose and gradually increase if needed. For children, the elderly, and pregnant or breastfeeding women, even smaller doses are recommended (see sections below).

---

4. Be Aware of Contraindications

A contraindication means that a certain herb should not be used in specific circumstances, such as when taking particular medications or dealing with certain health conditions.

Common Contraindications to Know

- **Pregnancy and Breastfeeding:** Some herbs, like pennyroyal or blue cohosh, can stimulate uterine contractions and should be avoided. Other herbs, like chamomile or nettle, are considered safe but should still be used in moderation.
- **Medication Interactions:**
  - **St. John's Wort** can interfere with antidepressants, blood thinners, and hormonal birth control.
  - **Ginkgo Biloba** may thin the blood and should be avoided if you're taking anticoagulants like warfarin.
  - **Licorice Root** can raise blood pressure and interact with diuretics.
- **Chronic Conditions:**
  - People with liver or kidney conditions should be cautious with herbs like comfrey or kava, which can

stress these organs when used long-term.

- Diabetics should monitor blood sugar closely when using herbs like cinnamon or fenugreek, as they may lower glucose levels.

When in doubt, consult a healthcare professional or licensed herbalist before using a new herb, especially if you're taking prescription medications or have ongoing health concerns.

---

5. Special Considerations for Children

Herbs can be a wonderful way to support children's health, but their smaller bodies require smaller doses and extra care. Always use gentle herbs and age-appropriate preparations.

Child-Safe Herbs:

- **Chamomile:** Great for soothing tummy troubles or calming restlessness.
- **Elderflower:** Helpful for colds and fevers.
- **Peppermint:** A mild remedy for nausea or digestive discomfort.

Child Dosage Rule:

A common guideline is **Clark's Rule**, which calculates dosage based on a child's weight:

- Divide the child's weight (in pounds) by 150. Multiply that fraction by the adult dose.

For example, if a child weighs 50 pounds and the adult dose is 30 drops of tincture:
50 ÷ 150 = 1/3 of the adult dose = 10 drops.

---

6. Special Considerations for Pregnant and Nursing Women

Pregnancy and nursing are times of heightened sensitivity, and not all herbs are safe for use during these stages. Some herbs can stimulate uterine contractions, cross into breast milk, or affect hormonal balance.

Safe Herbs for Pregnancy:

- **Ginger:** Helps with nausea and morning sickness.
- **Raspberry Leaf:** Tones the uterus and prepares the body for labor (best used in the second and third trimesters).
- **Peppermint:** Relieves nausea and aids digestion.

Herbs to Avoid:

- **Pennyroyal**
- **Blue Cohosh**
- **Dong Quai**
- **Sage (in large amounts)**

Always consult with a midwife, herbalist, or healthcare provider before using herbs during pregnancy or while breastfeeding.

---

7. Foraging and Wildcrafting Safely

If you're interested in foraging for your own herbs, safety is paramount. Some plants have toxic lookalikes that can cause harm if misidentified.

Foraging Safety Tips:

- Use a trusted plant identification guide or app.

- Only harvest plants you're 100% certain of—when in doubt, leave it out.
- Avoid harvesting near roads, industrial areas, or places where pesticides or pollutants may be present.

---

8. Recognizing and Responding to Adverse Reactions

Though rare, adverse reactions to herbs can occur, especially in people with allergies or sensitivities. Here's what to look out for:

Common Signs of Adverse Reactions:

- Digestive upset (nausea, diarrhea, or cramps)
- Skin irritation (itching, redness, or rash)
- Difficulty breathing or swelling (a sign of a serious allergic reaction)

What to Do:

- **Mild Reactions:** Stop using the herb immediately and drink plenty of water. Symptoms often resolve on their own.
- **Severe Reactions:** If you experience difficulty breathing, swelling, or other signs of a severe allergic reaction, seek emergency medical care immediately.

---

9. When to Consult a Professional

While herbs are wonderful for everyday ailments and general wellness, some situations call for professional medical advice:

- Persistent or worsening symptoms.
- Severe pain, high fever, or other signs of serious illness.
- Uncertainty about herb-drug interactions or underlying

health conditions.

Herbs are a complementary tool, not a substitute for appropriate medical care.

---

10. Adopt a Mindful, Respectful Approach

Herbalism is as much about respecting nature as it is about healing. Practice sustainability and gratitude as you work with herbs:

- **Use ethically sourced herbs:** Buy from trusted suppliers or grow your own.
- **Harvest responsibly:** Take only what you need and leave enough for the plant to thrive.
- **Respect tradition:** Many herbal practices have deep cultural and spiritual significance. Approach this knowledge with gratitude and humility.

PART 1: FOUNDATIONS OF HERBAL HEALING

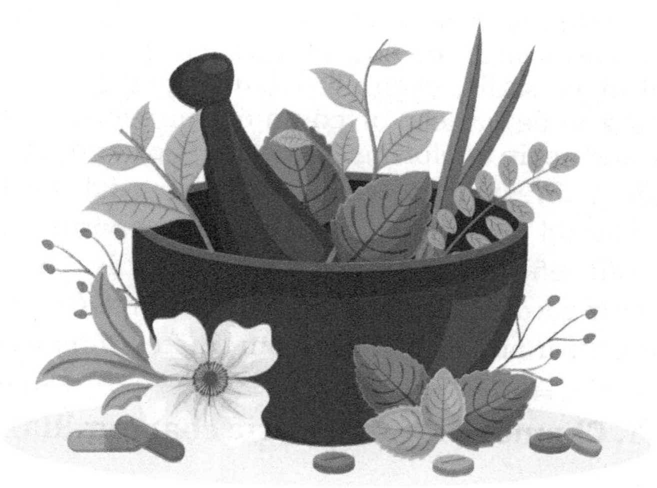

1.1 BUILDING YOUR HOME APOTHECARY

Starting your home apothecary can feel both exciting and overwhelming, but don't worry—you don't need to start with a full shelf of jars or dozens of herbs. With just a handful of versatile, beginner-friendly herbs, you'll be able to address a wide variety of common ailments, craft simple remedies, and begin exploring the healing power of plants.

This chapter introduces the **10–15 essential herbs** every beginner should consider for their home apothecary. These herbs are safe, effective, and incredibly versatile. You can grow them in your garden, forage them in your area (depending on your location), or purchase them from trusted suppliers.

---

1. Chamomile (Matricaria chamomilla)

The Soother

- **Uses:** Calms anxiety, promotes sleep, soothes upset stomachs, eases menstrual cramps, and reduces inflammation.
- **Best Forms:** Dried flowers (for teas, compresses, or infusions).
- **Why It's Essential:** Chamomile is gentle enough for children yet effective for adults. Its calming properties make it invaluable for stress relief, and it's a must-have for anyone dealing with sleep issues.

- **Quick Recipe:** Steep 1–2 teaspoons of dried chamomile flowers in hot water for 10 minutes to make a calming tea.

---

2. Peppermint (Mentha × piperita)

The Energizer

- **Uses:** Eases digestive discomfort, relieves headaches, clears sinuses, and boosts energy.
- **Best Forms:** Fresh or dried leaves (for teas, infusions, or compresses); peppermint essential oil (for aromatherapy or topical use).
- **Why It's Essential:** Peppermint's cooling and invigorating properties make it a go-to remedy for bloating, nausea, and fatigue. It's also fantastic for clearing the mind.
- **Quick Recipe:** Place fresh or dried peppermint leaves in boiling water to create a refreshing digestive tea.

---

3. Lavender (Lavandula angustifolia)

The Relaxer

- **Uses:** Relieves stress and anxiety, promotes restful sleep, soothes burns and insect bites, and reduces headaches.
- **Best Forms:** Dried flowers (for teas, sachets, or baths); lavender essential oil (for aromatherapy or skin applications).
- **Why It's Essential:** Lavender is a multipurpose herb for emotional wellness and skincare. Its soothing scent and anti-inflammatory properties make it a staple in any apothecary.
- **Quick Recipe:** Add a handful of dried lavender flowers to a

warm bath for a relaxing soak.

---

4. Calendula (Calendula officinalis)

The Healer

- **Uses:** Treats cuts, scrapes, rashes, burns, and minor skin irritations; promotes wound healing; and soothes inflamed skin.
- **Best Forms:** Dried petals (for salves, oils, and teas).
- **Why It's Essential:** Calendula is the ultimate skin healer. Its antimicrobial and anti-inflammatory properties make it perfect for DIY salves and creams.
- **Quick Recipe:** Infuse calendula petals in olive oil and use the oil as a base for homemade salves.

---

5. Ginger (Zingiber officinale)

The Warmer

- **Uses:** Relieves nausea, soothes sore throats, improves digestion, and fights inflammation.
- **Best Forms:** Fresh root (for teas, syrups, or cooking); dried powder (for capsules or teas).
- **Why It's Essential:** Ginger is warming and energizing, making it perfect for cold days, upset stomachs, or fighting off colds and flu.
- **Quick Recipe:** Simmer fresh ginger slices in water for 10 minutes to make a warming tea.

---

6. Echinacea (Echinacea purpurea)

The Immune Booster

- **Uses:** Supports the immune system, helps fight colds and flu, and speeds up recovery from illness.
- **Best Forms:** Dried root or flowers (for teas or tinctures).
- **Why It's Essential:** Echinacea is one of the most trusted herbs for immune health. It's especially useful during cold and flu season.
- **Quick Recipe:** Make a tincture by steeping echinacea root in vodka for 4–6 weeks. Take 1–2 droppers full at the first sign of a cold.

---

7. Elderberry (Sambucus nigra)

The Defender

- **Uses:** Boosts immunity, treats colds and flu, and reduces inflammation.
- **Best Forms:** Dried berries (for syrups, teas, or tinctures).
- **Why It's Essential:** Elderberry is a powerhouse for preventing and treating seasonal illnesses. Plus, it tastes delicious, making it great for kids.
- **Quick Recipe:** Simmer dried elderberries with honey and water to create a sweet, immune-boosting syrup.

---

8. Turmeric (Curcuma longa)

The Anti-Inflammatory

- **Uses:** Reduces inflammation, supports joint health, aids digestion, and promotes liver detoxification.
- **Best Forms:** Dried powder (for teas, capsules, or golden

milk); fresh root (for cooking or teas).

- **Why It's Essential:** Turmeric's anti-inflammatory properties make it essential for managing chronic pain, arthritis, or post-exercise recovery.
- **Quick Recipe:** Stir 1 teaspoon of turmeric powder into warm milk with a pinch of black pepper for a soothing golden milk.

---

9. Yarrow (Achillea millefolium)

The Protector

- **Uses:** Stops bleeding, reduces fevers, soothes digestive upset, and promotes wound healing.
- **Best Forms:** Dried flowers and leaves (for teas, poultices, or salves).
- **Why It's Essential:** Yarrow is a first-aid kit in a plant, perfect for scrapes, fevers, or inflammation.
- **Quick Recipe:** Make a yarrow poultice by crushing fresh leaves and applying them directly to wounds to stop bleeding.

---

10. Lemon Balm (Melissa officinalis)

The Uplifter

- **Uses:** Calms anxiety, improves mood, aids digestion, and supports restful sleep.
- **Best Forms:** Fresh or dried leaves (for teas or infusions).
- **Why It's Essential:** Lemon balm is gentle yet uplifting, making it perfect for both emotional and physical wellness.

- **Quick Recipe:** Brew a tea with lemon balm leaves to ease stress and brighten your day.

---

11. Dandelion (Taraxacum officinale)

The Detoxifier

- **Uses:** Supports liver health, aids digestion, reduces water retention, and provides gentle detoxification.
- **Best Forms:** Fresh or dried leaves and roots (for teas, infusions, or tinctures).
- **Why It's Essential:** Dandelion is a nutrient-rich herb that helps with cleansing and balancing the body.
- **Quick Recipe:** Brew the roasted root as a coffee substitute or make a tea from the leaves to support digestion.

---

12. Rosemary (Rosmarinus officinalis)

The Stimulator

- **Uses:** Enhances memory and focus, boosts circulation, soothes sore muscles, and promotes hair growth.
- **Best Forms:** Fresh or dried leaves (for teas, oils, or cooking).
- **Why It's Essential:** Rosemary is a kitchen staple with powerful cognitive and circulatory benefits, making it both useful and delicious.
- **Quick Recipe:** Infuse rosemary in olive oil for a multipurpose hair treatment or massage oil.

---

13. Cayenne Pepper (Capsicum annuum)

The Circulation Booster

- **Uses:** Stimulates circulation, relieves pain, and clears sinus congestion.
- **Best Forms:** Dried powder (for teas, salves, or poultices).
- **Why It's Essential:** Cayenne adds warmth to any remedy, making it excellent for boosting blood flow and easing aches.
- **Quick Recipe:** Add a pinch of cayenne powder to warm water and honey to create a natural decongestant.

---

14. Slippery Elm (Ulmus rubra)

The Soother

- **Uses:** Coats and soothes sore throats, eases digestive irritation, and promotes healing of the gut lining.
- **Best Forms:** Powdered inner bark (for teas or pastes).
- **Why It's Essential:** Slippery elm is a gentle, soothing herb, perfect for sore throats or stomach irritation.
- **Quick Recipe:** Mix slippery elm powder with warm water and honey to create a soothing throat paste.

---

15. Thyme (Thymus vulgaris)

The Antimicrobial

- **Uses:** Treats colds, clears respiratory congestion, and fights bacterial and fungal infections.
- **Best Forms:** Fresh or dried leaves (for teas, steams, or gargles).
- **Why It's Essential:** Thyme is a natural antibiotic and a go-to

herb for respiratory and immune support.

- **Quick Recipe:** Make a thyme tea to soothe coughs and support respiratory health.

Final Thoughts

With these 10–15 herbs, you'll have a versatile foundation for your home apothecary. They're beginner-friendly, widely available, and can address a wide range of common health concerns. As you grow more confident, you can begin exploring additional herbs and remedies to expand your collection.

In the next section, we'll cover the tools, jars, and ingredients you'll need to store and prepare these herbs—because every great apothecary needs a little organization and care!

1.2 ESSENTIAL TOOLS AND INGREDIENTS

Building a home apothecary is a rewarding journey, and like any craft, it starts with having the right tools and ingredients. While herbal remedies can often be made with just a few simple items you already have in your kitchen, investing in a few key tools will make the process easier, more efficient, and more enjoyable.

This chapter covers the essential tools and ingredients every beginner needs to create herbal teas, tinctures, salves, and more. We'll also walk you through the basic preparations step by step so you can start crafting remedies right away.

Essential Tools for Your Home Apothecary

The following tools are practical, easy to find, and versatile enough to handle a wide variety of herbal preparations.

1. Jars and Containers

You'll need jars of various sizes for storing herbs, oils, and finished remedies. Look for glass containers with tight-fitting lids to preserve freshness and potency.

- **Mason jars**: Perfect for infusions, tinctures, and herbal oils.
- **Small jars or tins**: Ideal for salves, balms, and creams.
- **Amber or cobalt bottles**: Great for tinctures and essential oil blends to protect them from light.

2. Strainers and Cheesecloth

You'll need something to strain herbs from liquids when making teas, tinctures, and oils.

- **Fine-mesh strainers**: Handy for separating herbs from teas and infusions.
- **Cheesecloth or muslin bags**: Great for squeezing every last drop from infused oils or tinctures.

3. Mortar and Pestle or Grinder

A mortar and pestle is a classic tool for grinding dried herbs into powders or breaking down fresh herbs. For larger quantities, a **coffee or spice grinder** works well for dried herbs.

4. Measuring Tools

- **Measuring cups and spoons**: To ensure consistent dosages.
- **Kitchen scale**: For weighing herbs, especially when working with larger recipes.

5. Double Boiler or Heatproof Bowl

When making salves, balms, or herbal oils, a double boiler ensures gentle, even heating without overheating your ingredients. If you don't have one, you can use a heatproof bowl over a pot of simmering water.

6. Funnels

A small funnel makes it easy to transfer tinctures, oils, and salves into jars and bottles without spilling.

7. Labels and Markers

Label every jar, bottle, and tin with the name of the remedy, the ingredients, and the date it was made. You'll thank yourself later when you're not guessing what's inside!

8. Spray Bottles and Droppers

- **Spray bottles**: Perfect for herbal mists, toners, and room sprays.
- **Dropper bottles**: Ideal for tinctures, glycerites, or essential oil blends.

Essential Ingredients for Your Home Apothecary

In addition to the herbs themselves, there are a few basic ingredients that you'll use repeatedly in your remedies:

1. Carrier Oils

Carrier oils are the base for salves, balms, and infused oils. They nourish the skin and allow you to extract the active properties of herbs.

- **Olive oil**: Versatile and great for most skin types.
- **Coconut oil**: Ideal for balms, thanks to its solid texture at room temperature.
- **Sweet almond oil**: Lightweight and excellent for sensitive skin.
- **Jojoba oil**: Long shelf life and non-greasy; perfect for facial care.

2. Beeswax or Plant-Based Waxes

Beeswax is used to thicken balms and salves. For a vegan alternative, try **carnauba wax** or **candelilla wax**.

3. Alcohol for Tinctures

High-proof alcohol (like vodka, brandy, or grain alcohol) is used to extract and preserve the medicinal properties of herbs in tinctures. Choose a clear alcohol that's at least 40% alcohol (80 proof).

4. Vinegar

Apple cider vinegar is a great alternative to alcohol for making tinctures, especially for children or those who avoid alcohol.

5. Honey

Honey is often used in syrups and teas for its soothing and antimicrobial properties. It also acts as a natural preservative.

6. Shea Butter or Cocoa Butter

Rich and nourishing, these butters are fantastic for creating skin-healing salves and balms.

7. Distilled Water

Distilled water is free of impurities and ideal for herbal teas, facial steams, and sprays.

8. Essential Oils

A small collection of essential oils adds fragrance and therapeutic properties to your remedies. Start with a few versatile options, such as lavender, peppermint, tea tree, and eucalyptus.

Simple Preparations: Teas, Tinctures, Salves, and More

Step-by-Step Tutorials for Creating Basic Remedies

Now that you have your tools and ingredients ready, let's dive into the basics of herbal preparation. These methods are the foundation of your home apothecary and will allow you to craft a wide range of remedies.

---

1. Herbal Teas (Infusions and Decoctions)

Infusion (for leaves, flowers, and soft parts of herbs)

Infusions are the easiest way to extract the medicinal properties of soft herbs like chamomile, peppermint, and lemon balm.

What You'll Need:

- 1–2 teaspoons dried herbs (or 1 tablespoon fresh herbs)
- 1 cup boiling water

Steps:

1. Place the herbs in a teapot or heatproof mug.
2. Pour boiling water over the herbs.
3. Cover and let steep for 5–15 minutes. (Longer steeping extracts more medicinal compounds.)
4. Strain and enjoy. Add honey or lemon if desired.

Decoction (for roots, bark, and tough herbs)

Decoctions are used for harder herbs like ginger, licorice root, or cinnamon sticks.

What You'll Need:

- 1 tablespoon dried roots or bark
- 1 cup water

Steps:

1. Add the herbs and water to a small pot.

2. Bring to a boil, then reduce heat and simmer for 15–30 minutes.
3. Strain and enjoy.

---

2. Tinctures

Tinctures are potent, concentrated extracts made by steeping herbs in alcohol or vinegar.

What You'll Need:

- Dried or fresh herbs (cut into small pieces)
- High-proof alcohol (like vodka)
- Mason jar with lid

Steps:

1. Fill a clean jar halfway with herbs.
2. Pour alcohol over the herbs until completely submerged, leaving about 1 inch of space at the top.
3. Seal the jar tightly and shake well.
4. Store in a cool, dark place for 4–6 weeks, shaking the jar every few days.
5. Strain the mixture through cheesecloth or a fine-mesh strainer into a dropper bottle.
6. Label the tincture with the herb name and date.

Dosage: Typically, 20–40 drops diluted in water, 1–3 times daily.

---

3. Salves and Balms

Salves are soothing ointments made by combining infused oils with beeswax. They're perfect for cuts, burns, rashes, and dry skin.

What You'll Need:

- Herbal-infused oil (e.g., calendula, lavender, or comfrey oil)
- Beeswax
- Double boiler

Steps:

1. Measure 1/4 cup of infused oil and 1 tablespoon of beeswax.
2. Melt the beeswax in a double boiler over low heat.
3. Add the infused oil and stir until combined.
4. Remove from heat and pour into tins or small jars.
5. Let cool until solid, then cover and label.

---

4. Herbal Syrups

Syrups are sweet, soothing remedies perfect for colds, coughs, and sore throats.

What You'll Need:

- 1 cup dried herbs (like elderberries or licorice root)
- 4 cups water
- 1 cup honey

Steps:

1. Combine herbs and water in a pot and bring to a boil.
2. Reduce heat and simmer until the liquid is reduced by half

(about 20–30 minutes).

3. Strain the mixture and let it cool slightly.
4. Stir in honey until fully dissolved.
5. Pour into a glass jar and store in the fridge for up to 1 month.

Dosage: 1–2 teaspoons, 2–3 times daily.

Final Thoughts

With just a few tools, ingredients, and these simple techniques, you'll be able to create teas, tinctures, salves, and syrups to support your health naturally. These preparations form the foundation of your herbal apothecary, allowing you to craft remedies for common ailments with ease.

As you practice these methods, you'll build confidence and start to develop your own style of herbal crafting. Remember, herbalism is a creative and personal journey—have fun experimenting and enjoy the process!

In the next section, we'll dive deeper into understanding herbs and their unique properties, helping you customize remedies for your specific needs. Let's continue!

1.3 UNDERSTANDING HERBS AND THEIR ENERGETICS

Herbalism isn't just about the properties of individual plants (like "anti-inflammatory" or "immune-boosting"). It's also about understanding how herbs interact with the body's natural state and balance. This is where the concept of herbal energetics comes in—a way to understand how herbs influence the body's internal environment.

In herbalism, the body's health is often viewed in terms of balance. Is your body running too hot, too cold, too dry, or too damp? Understanding your body's tendencies, combined with the energetics of herbs, allows you to choose the right remedy to restore balance and promote healing.

This chapter will guide you through the basics of herbal energetics, introduce you to cooling, warming, moistening, and drying herbs, and teach you how to match the right herb to your body's specific needs.

What Are Herbal Energetics?

Herbal energetics is an ancient concept rooted in traditional systems of medicine like Ayurveda, Traditional Chinese Medicine (TCM), and Western herbalism. It describes the **effect an herb has on the body's internal state**, helping to restore harmony where imbalance exists.

At its core, herbal energetics is about the qualities of herbs and how they interact with the body. The four main energetic qualities are:

- **Cooling vs. Warming**: Does the herb help cool down or warm up the body?
- **Moistening vs. Drying**: Does the herb increase moisture or reduce dampness?

These qualities are essential because many ailments have an energetic component. For example:

- A fever is a "hot" condition that benefits from cooling herbs.
- Dry, irritated skin is a "dry" condition that benefits from moistening herbs.
- Cold, sluggish digestion is a "cold" condition that benefits from warming herbs.
- Excess mucus or swelling is a "damp" condition that benefits from drying herbs.

By understanding both your body's energetic state and the energetics of herbs, you can tailor remedies for more effective healing.

Cooling Herbs

For Overheated or Inflamed Conditions

Cooling herbs help reduce excess heat in the body. They are often used for fevers, hot flashes, inflammation, rashes, and conditions where there's redness, irritation, or a "burning" sensation.

When to Use Cooling Herbs:

- Fever or heat-related illness.
- Inflammation (like swollen joints or irritated skin).

- Stress or anxiety that feels agitating or fiery.
- Heat-related digestive issues like acid reflux.

Examples of Cooling Herbs:

- **Peppermint**: A classic cooling herb for fevers, headaches, and hot flashes.
- **Chamomile**: Gently cools inflammation and calms an overheated nervous system.
- **Elderflower**: Reduces fever and supports the body during colds or flu.
- **Lemon Balm**: Soothes anxiety and cools an overactive mind.
- **Cucumber and Aloe Vera**: External cooling herbs for burns and irritated skin.

Warming Herbs

For Cold, Sluggish, or Stagnant Conditions

Warming herbs increase circulation, stimulate digestion, and bring warmth to cold areas of the body. They are perfect for chilly winter days, sluggish digestion, poor circulation, or cold hands and feet.

When to Use Warming Herbs:

- Cold, stagnant digestion (bloating, gas, or a heavy feeling after meals).
- Cold hands and feet or poor circulation.
- Feeling tired, lethargic, or "stuck."
- Coughs with thin, clear mucus.

Examples of Warming Herbs:

- **Ginger**: A powerhouse for warming digestion, boosting circulation, and easing nausea.
- **Cinnamon**: Warms the body, regulates blood sugar, and supports the respiratory system.
- **Garlic**: Stimulates circulation and boosts the immune system.
- **Cayenne Pepper**: Provides an instant warming boost, relieves pain, and clears sinuses.
- **Clove**: A warming herb for sore throats and cold-related aches.

Moistening Herbs

For Dry, Irritated, or Dehydrated Conditions

Moistening herbs restore hydration to tissues that are dry, inflamed, or irritated. They are often used for dry skin, dry coughs, constipation, or dryness in the throat and digestive tract.

When to Use Moistening Herbs:

- Dry, hacking coughs.
- Dry skin or chapped lips.
- Constipation caused by dryness.
- A dry, irritated throat or mouth.

Examples of Moistening Herbs:

- **Marshmallow Root**: Soothes dry coughs, sore throats, and irritated digestive tissues.

- **Slippery Elm**: Protects and hydrates the throat, stomach lining, and intestines.
- **Licorice Root**: Hydrates tissues and reduces inflammation in the respiratory and digestive systems.
- **Oats (Milky Oat Tops)**: Nourish and moisturize the nervous system, easing stress and dryness.
- **Chia Seeds**: Hydrating when soaked; excellent for internal dryness and constipation.

Drying Herbs

For Damp, Mucusy, or Swollen Conditions

Drying herbs reduce excess moisture, dampness, and mucus in the body. They are useful for conditions like sinus congestion, wet coughs, swelling, or sluggish digestion.

When to Use Drying Herbs:

- Congestion or excess mucus (e.g., sinus infections or wet coughs).
- Damp, swollen tissues.
- Loose stools or diarrhea.
- Digestive issues related to excess moisture.

Examples of Drying Herbs:

- **Sage**: Dries up excess mucus, soothes sore throats, and reduces sweating.
- **Yarrow**: Balances damp conditions and supports wound healing.
- **Thyme**: Dries mucus, treats respiratory infections, and acts

as a natural antimicrobial.

- **Rosemary**: Stimulates digestion and reduces dampness in the body.
- **Horsetail**: A diuretic herb that dries and tones tissues, often used for urinary health.

How to Choose the Right Herb for Your Body

When selecting an herb, consider two key factors:

1. **Your Body's State:** Is your body too hot, too cold, too dry, or too damp?
    - Example: A fever is hot, so you'd choose cooling herbs like peppermint or elderflower.
    - Example: A dry, hacking cough benefits from moistening herbs like marshmallow root or slippery elm.
    - Example: A wet cough with thick mucus calls for drying herbs like thyme or sage.
2. **The Herb's Energetics:** Does the herb cool, warm, moisten, or dry? Match the herb's qualities to the condition you're treating.

Combining Energetics for a Balanced Remedy

Often, you'll need to balance multiple energetics in a remedy. For example:

- **Cough Remedy:** If a cough is dry and irritated, combine moistening (marshmallow root) and cooling (peppermint) herbs.

- **Cold and Flu Remedy:** If you have chills and body aches, use warming (ginger) and drying (sage) herbs to improve circulation and reduce mucus.
- **Digestive Remedy:** For bloating and gas (cold and damp), combine warming (cinnamon) and drying (rosemary) herbs.

Experiment with blending herbs to create remedies that are customized to your unique needs.

Final Thoughts

Understanding herbal energetics is like learning a new language—it opens up a deeper relationship with plants and your body. By tuning into your body's natural state and learning how to choose herbs that balance your specific needs, you'll take your herbal practice to the next level.

As you work with herbs, you'll begin to notice patterns: which herbs feel cooling, which feel warming, and how your body responds to each one. Over time, this knowledge will empower you to craft remedies that are not only effective but truly personalized.

In the next section, we'll explore **herbal actions** (like anti-inflammatory, adaptogenic, and antimicrobial) to give you even more tools for understanding how herbs work. Let's continue!

1.4 HERBAL ACTIONS: ANTI-INFLAMMATORY, ADAPTOGENIC, ANTIMICROBIAL

As you begin working with herbs, you'll encounter terms that describe their actions, or how they influence the body. Herbal actions are a way of categorizing herbs by their effects, making it easier to choose the right one for a specific purpose.

This chapter will break down some of the most common herbal actions—like **anti-inflammatory**, **adaptogenic**, and **antimicrobial**—and show you how to use them in everyday health. You'll also learn how to combine herbs to create synergistic blends that enhance their effectiveness.

What Are Herbal Actions?

Herbal actions describe what an herb *does*. For example, an herb that reduces swelling and pain is said to have an anti-inflammatory action. Many herbs have multiple actions, which is why they can be so versatile.

Knowing these actions will help you make informed choices when building remedies. Let's explore three key herbal actions that you'll use again and again:

---

1. Anti-Inflammatory Herbs

Reducing Inflammation for Pain Relief and Healing

Inflammation is a natural part of the body's healing process, but chronic inflammation can lead to pain, swelling, and long-term health issues like arthritis, heart disease, or autoimmune conditions. Anti-inflammatory herbs can help reduce inflammation gently and effectively.

When to Use Anti-Inflammatory Herbs:

- To relieve pain from sore muscles, joint stiffness, or arthritis.
- To soothe digestive inflammation, like gastritis or IBS.
- For skin conditions like eczema, rashes, or wounds.

Examples of Anti-Inflammatory Herbs:

- **Turmeric:** Reduces inflammation in joints and supports overall immune health.
- **Ginger:** Calms digestive inflammation and helps reduce muscle soreness.
- **Chamomile:** Soothes irritated tissues and eases digestive discomfort.
- **Calendula:** Reduces skin inflammation and promotes wound healing.
- **Willow Bark:** A natural pain reliever and anti-inflammatory (the precursor to aspirin).

Quick Remedy Idea:

Anti-Inflammatory Tea for Pain Relief

- 1 tsp dried turmeric
- 1 tsp dried ginger
- 1 tsp chamomile flowers
- Steep in hot water for 10 minutes. Strain and enjoy up to 3 times a day.

---

2. Adaptogenic Herbs

Helping the Body Adapt to Stress and Build Resilience

Adaptogens are herbs that help the body adapt to physical, mental, and emotional stress. They work by regulating the adrenal glands, supporting hormonal balance, and boosting energy levels. These herbs are best taken regularly over time for long-term benefits.

When to Use Adaptogenic Herbs:

- To reduce chronic stress and fatigue.
- To improve focus, endurance, and energy levels.
- To balance hormones and support overall resilience.

Examples of Adaptogenic Herbs:

- **Ashwagandha:** Reduces stress, supports sleep, and strengthens the immune system.
- **Holy Basil (Tulsi):** Promotes mental clarity and emotional balance.
- **Rhodiola:** Increases stamina and reduces fatigue.
- **Eleuthero (Siberian Ginseng):** Boosts energy and improves focus.

- **Reishi Mushroom:** Supports immune health and emotional well-being.

Quick Remedy Idea:

Morning Adaptogen Tonic for Energy and Focus

- 1 tsp powdered ashwagandha
- 1 tsp powdered reishi mushroom
- 1 cup warm almond milk
- 1 tsp honey (optional)
- Mix well and drink in the morning for sustained energy.

---

3. Antimicrobial Herbs

Fighting Infections and Supporting Immunity

Antimicrobial herbs help fight bacteria, viruses, and fungi. They're excellent for preventing and treating colds, flu, skin infections, and digestive imbalances. Unlike synthetic antibiotics, antimicrobial herbs typically support the body's natural microbiome without destroying beneficial bacteria.

When to Use Antimicrobial Herbs:

- For colds, sore throats, and respiratory infections.
- To treat skin infections or wounds.
- For digestive infections or imbalances.

Examples of Antimicrobial Herbs:

- **Garlic:** A natural antibiotic and antifungal herb.
- **Thyme:** Excellent for respiratory infections and sore

throats.

- **Oregano:** A powerful antiviral and antibacterial herb.
- **Echinacea:** Boosts the immune system and helps fight off infections.
- **Goldenseal:** Combats bacterial infections and supports mucous membrane health.

Quick Remedy Idea:

Antimicrobial Throat Gargle for Sore Throats

- 1 cup warm water
- 1 tsp dried thyme
- 1 tsp salt
- Steep the thyme in hot water for 10 minutes. Strain, add salt, and gargle 2–3 times a day.

Combining Herbs for Maximum Effectiveness

The Basics of Creating Synergistic Blends

Herbs often work better together. By combining herbs with complementary actions, you can create remedies that address multiple aspects of a condition while enhancing the effectiveness of each herb. This is called **synergy**.

Key Tips for Creating Synergistic Herbal Blends:

1. **Choose a Primary Herb (the Star):**
   Start by selecting one herb that addresses the main concern. For example:
   - **Turmeric** for inflammation.

- **Peppermint** for digestive discomfort.
- **Ashwagandha** for stress and fatigue.

2. **Add Supporting Herbs (the Helpers):**
Select 1–2 herbs that enhance or complement the primary herb's action. For example:
    - Add **ginger** to turmeric to boost anti-inflammatory effects.
    - Combine **fennel** with peppermint for additional digestive soothing.
    - Blend **holy basil** with ashwagandha to create a balanced adaptogenic blend.
3. **Include a Balancing Herb (the Harmonizer):**
Harmonizing herbs make a blend more palatable or add a touch of additional support. For example:
    - Add **chamomile** for a calming effect and a pleasant flavor.
    - Use **licorice root** to sweeten and balance a strong-tasting tea.

Example: Creating a Synergistic Blend

Blend for Cold and Flu Relief:

Primary Herb: Elderberry (to boost immunity and fight infection).
Supporting Herbs: Ginger (to warm the body and reduce inflammation) + Echinacea (to strengthen the immune response).
Balancing Herb: Peppermint (to soothe congestion and add a refreshing flavor).

Recipe:

- 1 part dried elderberries
- 1 part dried echinacea root
- 1/2 part dried ginger root
- 1/2 part dried peppermint leaves
  Mix all ingredients in a jar. To prepare, steep 1 tablespoon of the blend in 1 cup of boiling water for 10–15 minutes. Strain and enjoy 2–3 times daily.

Common Synergistic Pairings

- **Anti-Inflammatory Duo:** Turmeric + Ginger.
- **Stress Relief Duo:** Ashwagandha + Holy Basil.
- **Immune Booster Trio:** Elderberry + Echinacea + Thyme.
- **Digestive Soother:** Peppermint + Fennel.
- **Sleep Support:** Chamomile + Lemon Balm.

PART 2: REMEDIES FOR EVERYDAY AILMENTS

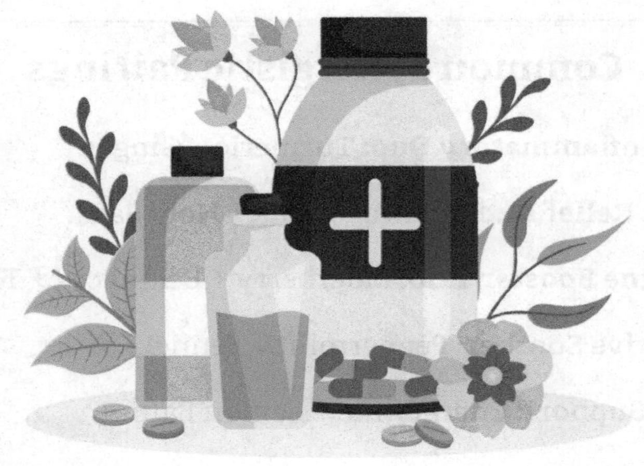

2.1 RESPIRATORY SUPPORT

The respiratory system is often the first to be affected by seasonal changes, colds, flu, and allergies. Herbs can play a vital role in easing symptoms like coughing, congestion, sneezing, and shortness of breath, while also supporting the immune system and reducing inflammation.

Remedies for Coughs, Colds, and Congestion

1. Elderberry and Echinacea Immune Tea

- Combine 1 teaspoon each of dried elderberries and echinacea in 1 cup boiling water.
- Steep for 10 minutes, strain, and drink 2–3 times daily.
- Supports immunity and reduces the duration of colds.

2. Ginger and Honey Cough Syrup

- Simmer 1/4 cup fresh ginger slices in 2 cups water until reduced by half.
- Strain and mix with 1/2 cup honey. Take 1 teaspoon every few hours to soothe coughs.

3. Peppermint Steam for Chest Congestion

- Add 1 tablespoon dried peppermint leaves (or 2 drops peppermint essential oil) to a bowl of hot water.
- Inhale deeply to open airways and reduce congestion.

4. Mullein Tea for Cough and Mucus

- Steep 1 teaspoon dried mullein leaves in 1 cup boiling water for 10 minutes.
- Strain through a fine mesh to remove hairs, and drink 2–3 times daily.

5. Thyme and Garlic Respiratory Tonic

- Infuse 1 teaspoon dried thyme and 1 crushed garlic clove in 1 cup boiling water.
- Strain, sweeten with honey, and sip to clear congestion and support respiratory health.

6. Onion and Honey Cough Remedy

- Slice a raw onion and layer it in a jar with honey.
- Let sit overnight and use the syrup to calm coughs (1 teaspoon as needed).

7. Elecampane Root Decoction

- Simmer 1 tablespoon dried elecampane root in 2 cups water for 15–20 minutes.
- Strain and sip throughout the day to relieve deep chest coughs.

8. Eucalyptus and Lavender Chest Rub

- Mix 1/4 cup coconut oil with 10 drops eucalyptus and 10 drops lavender essential oils.
- Massage onto the chest to ease breathing and relax the lungs.

9. Sage Gargle for Sore Throats and Coughs

- Steep 1 teaspoon dried sage in 1 cup hot water for 10 minutes.
- Add a pinch of salt and gargle 2–3 times a day to soothe a sore throat.

10. Lemon Balm Tea for Cold Relief

- Steep 1 teaspoon dried lemon balm leaves in hot water for 10 minutes.
- Drink to reduce stress, soothe coughing, and boost immunity.

11. Horseradish Paste for Stuffy Nose

- Grate fresh horseradish root and mix with a little apple cider vinegar.
- Take a small amount (1/2 teaspoon) to promote sinus drainage.

12. Fire Cider for Cold and Congestion

- Combine apple cider vinegar with grated ginger, garlic, horseradish, and honey in a jar. Let it steep for 2 weeks, strain, and take 1 tablespoon daily.

13. Ginger and Turmeric Cold Tea

- Boil 1 teaspoon each of fresh grated ginger and turmeric in 2 cups water.
- Add honey and lemon for a warming, immune-boosting drink.

14. Elderberry Lozenges

- Simmer elderberry syrup with a little honey and gelatin, pour into molds, and let cool to form soothing cough drops.

15. Chamomile Tea for Mucus Reduction

- Steep 1 teaspoon chamomile in boiling water and sip to reduce inflammation and thin mucus.

16. Licorice Root Tea for Persistent Coughs

- Simmer 1 tablespoon licorice root in 2 cups water for 10 minutes.
- Strain and drink to ease coughing and throat irritation.

17. Fenugreek Seeds for Stubborn Mucus

- Simmer 1 tablespoon fenugreek seeds in 2 cups water for 10 minutes.
- Drink to reduce phlegm and congestion.

18. Garlic and Thyme Steam Inhalation

- Add crushed garlic and dried thyme to a bowl of steaming water.
- Inhale deeply to open airways and fight infections.

19. Turmeric Golden Milk for Inflammation

- Heat 1 cup milk (dairy or plant-based) with 1/2 teaspoon turmeric powder and a pinch of black pepper.
- Drink at bedtime for soothing relief from inflammation and coughing.

20. Pine Needle Tea for Lung Support

- Steep fresh pine needles in hot water for 10 minutes.
- Strain and drink to detoxify the lungs and strengthen respiratory function.

Herbal Relief for Seasonal Allergies

21. Nettle and Peppermint Tea for Hay Fever

- Combine 1 teaspoon each of dried nettle and peppermint in 1 cup boiling water.
- Steep for 10 minutes, strain, and drink to reduce sneezing and congestion.

22. Elderflower Infusion for Runny Nose

- Steep 1 tablespoon elderflowers in 1 cup boiling water for 15 minutes.
- Drink 1–2 cups daily to relieve nasal symptoms.

23. Quercetin-Rich Onion Broth

- Simmer onions, garlic, and a pinch of cayenne in water to create a simple broth.
- Sip to reduce histamine reactions and strengthen immunity.

24. Local Honey for Allergy Desensitization

- Take 1 teaspoon of raw, local honey daily to help the body adjust to local pollen.

25. Chamomile Compress for Itchy Eyes

- Steep chamomile tea bags in hot water, let cool, and place over the eyes for 10 minutes.

26. Butterbur Capsules for Seasonal Allergies

- Butterbur (available in capsule form) is an herbal antihistamine that reduces sneezing and nasal congestion.

27. Eucalyptus and Rosemary Steam

- Add eucalyptus and rosemary essential oils to a bowl of steaming water.
- Inhale to reduce sinus pressure and clear nasal passages.

28. Goldenrod Tea for Congestion

- Steep 1 teaspoon dried goldenrod in hot water for 10 minutes.
- Drink to reduce congestion and sinus pressure.

29. Apple Cider Vinegar Allergy Tonic

- Mix 1 tablespoon apple cider vinegar, 1 teaspoon honey, and warm water.
- Drink daily during allergy season to reduce symptoms.

30. Turmeric and Ginger Anti-Inflammatory Tea

- Combine 1/2 teaspoon turmeric, 1/2 teaspoon grated ginger, and a pinch of black pepper in hot water.
- Sip to calm inflammation and reduce allergy-related swelling.

2.2 DIGESTIVE WELLNESS

The digestive system is at the center of our overall health and wellness. Herbs can be a wonderful, natural way to soothe digestive discomforts, support gut health, and restore balance.

Solutions for Bloating, Nausea, and Indigestion

1. Peppermint Tea for Bloating

- Steep 1 teaspoon dried peppermint leaves in 1 cup boiling water for 10 minutes.
- Drink after meals to relieve gas, bloating, and stomach cramping.

2. Ginger Chews for Nausea Relief

- Peel and thinly slice fresh ginger.
- Simmer in a small amount of honey and water until soft, then let cool.
- Chew on a piece as needed to ease nausea and motion sickness.

3. Fennel Seed Tea for Gas and Cramping

- Crush 1 teaspoon fennel seeds and steep in 1 cup boiling water for 10 minutes.

- Drink to reduce gas, improve digestion, and ease abdominal pain.

4. Lemon and Honey Digestive Tonic

- Mix the juice of 1/2 lemon with 1 teaspoon honey in a cup of warm water.
- Sip slowly before or after meals to stimulate digestion and prevent indigestion.

5. Caraway Seed Infusion for Bloating

- Steep 1 teaspoon caraway seeds in 1 cup boiling water for 10 minutes.
- Strain and drink to ease bloating and flatulence.

6. Chamomile Tea for Upset Stomach

- Brew 1 teaspoon dried chamomile flowers in boiling water for 10 minutes.
- Drink to relax the digestive system and ease nausea or cramping.

7. Digestive Bitters Before Meals

- Take 1 teaspoon of an herbal digestive bitters blend (commercial or homemade) 10 minutes before meals to support healthy digestion and reduce bloating.

8. Cumin and Coriander Digestive Spice Tea

- Simmer 1/2 teaspoon each of cumin and coriander seeds in 2 cups water for 10 minutes.
- Strain and drink after meals to improve digestion and ease gas.

9. Apple Cider Vinegar Digestive Aid

- Mix 1 tablespoon apple cider vinegar in a cup of warm water.
- Drink before meals to stimulate digestion and prevent heartburn.

10. Dill Seed Tea for Stomach Discomfort

- Steep 1 teaspoon dill seeds in hot water for 10 minutes.
- Drink to relieve indigestion, nausea, and flatulence.

Gut-Healing Teas and Tonics

11. Marshmallow Root Tea for Gut Lining Repair

- Simmer 1 tablespoon dried marshmallow root in 2 cups water for 15 minutes.
- Strain and sip throughout the day to soothe inflammation and support the gut lining.

12. Slippery Elm Bark Infusion

- Mix 1 tablespoon slippery elm bark powder with 1 cup warm water.
- Stir until smooth and drink to coat and soothe the stomach and intestines.

13. Licorice Root Tea for Gut Health

- Simmer 1 teaspoon dried licorice root in 2 cups water for 10 minutes.
- Drink to reduce inflammation and support the healing of stomach ulcers.

14. Aloe Vera Juice for Digestive Comfort

- Mix 2 tablespoons pure aloe vera juice with 1/2 cup water or herbal tea.
- Drink to soothe irritation in the stomach and intestines.

15. Calendula Tea for Inflammation

- Steep 1 tablespoon dried calendula petals in hot water for 10 minutes.
- Drink to reduce gut inflammation and promote healing.

16. Turmeric and Ginger Gut-Healing Tonic

- Simmer 1 teaspoon turmeric powder and 1 teaspoon fresh grated ginger in 2 cups water.
- Add honey and sip to reduce inflammation and support the gut lining.

17. Nettle Tea for Gut Repair

- Steep 1 tablespoon dried nettle leaves in 2 cups boiling water for 10 minutes.
- Drink daily to nourish the gut and reduce inflammation.

18. Bone Broth Infused with Herbal Spices

- Simmer bone broth with ginger, garlic, and turmeric.
- Drink as a nourishing tonic to support gut health and heal the intestinal lining.

19. Oat and Licorice Soothing Drink

- Steep 1 tablespoon rolled oats and 1 teaspoon licorice root in 1 cup boiling water.

- Strain, sweeten with honey, and drink to calm gut irritation.

20. Cinnamon and Honey Digestive Support Tea

- Simmer 1 cinnamon stick in 2 cups water for 10 minutes.
- Add honey and drink to improve digestion and support a healthy gut microbiome.

Herbal Blends and Recipes for Digestive Wellness

21. Digestive Soother Herbal Blend

- Combine equal parts chamomile, fennel, and peppermint.
- Steep 1 teaspoon of the blend in 1 cup boiling water for 10 minutes.
- Drink after meals to relieve bloating and indigestion.

22. Anti-Bloating Tea Blend

- Combine equal parts caraway seeds, ginger root, and dandelion leaf.
- Brew 1 teaspoon of the blend in hot water for 10 minutes and drink as needed.

23. Cooling Aloe and Cucumber Tonic

- Blend 1/4 cup cucumber slices with 2 tablespoons aloe vera juice and 1 cup water.
- Sip to cool inflammation and soothe the stomach.

24. Lemon Balm and Chamomile Calming Tea

- Steep 1 teaspoon each of lemon balm and chamomile in

boiling water.

- Drink before bed to relax the stomach and calm the nervous system.

25. Ginger and Lemon Digestive Shot

- Blend 1 tablespoon fresh ginger juice with the juice of 1 lemon.

- Sip this small but potent shot to jumpstart digestion and ease nausea.

26. Digestive Detox Tea with Dandelion Root

- Simmer 1 teaspoon dried dandelion root in 2 cups water for 15 minutes.
- Strain and drink to support liver detox and promote healthy digestion.

27. Mint and Coriander Leaf Water

- Crush fresh mint and coriander leaves and steep in cold water for 15 minutes.

- Strain and sip throughout the day to support digestion.

28. Holy Basil (Tulsi) Gut-Healing Tea

- Brew 1 teaspoon dried holy basil leaves in 1 cup boiling water.
- Drink daily to reduce stress-induced digestive issues and support gut health.

29. Cinnamon, Ginger, and Fennel Digestive Powder

- Combine equal parts ground cinnamon, ginger, and fennel.

- Mix 1/2 teaspoon of the powder into warm water or tea to improve digestion.

30. Herbal Yogurt Digestive Bowl

- Mix 1 cup plain yogurt with fresh mint, grated ginger, and a pinch of cinnamon.
- Eat as a snack to nourish the gut microbiome and soothe the stomach.

2.3 PAIN AND INFLAMATION RELIEF

Pain and inflammation can affect us in countless ways, from nagging headaches to stiff joints and achy muscles. At the same time, seasonal illnesses like colds and flu can put stress on the body, triggering immune responses that lead to inflammation. Herbs offer a gentle, effective way to reduce pain, support the immune system, and promote faster recovery.

Remedies for Headaches

1. Peppermint and Lavender Headache Balm

- Mix 1/4 cup coconut oil with 10 drops peppermint essential oil and 5 drops lavender essential oil.
- Massage onto temples, neck, and shoulders for tension relief.

2. Feverfew Tincture for Migraine Prevention

- Take 1 dropperful of feverfew tincture (available commercially) once daily to reduce the frequency of migraines.

3. Ginger Tea for Headache Relief

- Simmer 1 teaspoon grated fresh ginger in 2 cups water for 10 minutes.

- Strain and sip to reduce inflammation and ease headaches.

4. Chamomile and Mint Headache Tea

- Combine 1 teaspoon each of dried chamomile and peppermint in boiling water.
- Steep for 10 minutes, strain, and drink to relieve tension headaches.

5. Rosemary Steam for Sinus Headaches

- Add 1 tablespoon dried rosemary to a bowl of steaming water.
- Drape a towel over your head and inhale deeply to ease sinus pressure.

6. White Willow Bark Decoction for Pain

- Simmer 1 teaspoon white willow bark in 2 cups water for 15 minutes.
- Strain and drink to reduce headache pain. (This herb is a natural source of salicin, similar to aspirin.)

7. Magnesium-Rich Herbal Drink for Headache Prevention

- Combine 1 teaspoon dried nettle with 1 teaspoon dried oat straw.
- Steep in hot water for 15 minutes and drink to reduce headache frequency.

8. Lavender Eye Compress for Stress-Induced Headaches

- Soak a cloth in cooled lavender tea and place over your eyes for 10 minutes.
- Helps relax tension and reduce headache pain.

9. Clove and Cinnamon Headache Tea

- Steep 1 clove and 1 small cinnamon stick in boiling water for 10 minutes.
- Drink warm to ease inflammation and soothe headaches.

10. Valerian Root Tonic for Tension Headaches

- Take 1 dropperful of valerian root tincture in water before bed to relax muscles and reduce tension headaches.

Remedies for Sore Muscles

11. Arnica Massage Oil for Muscle Pain

- Infuse arnica flowers in olive oil for 4 weeks, then strain.
- Massage onto sore muscles to reduce inflammation and pain.

12. Epsom Salt and Rosemary Bath Soak

- Add 1 cup Epsom salts and 1 tablespoon dried rosemary to a warm bath.
- Soak for 20 minutes to relax sore muscles.

13. Ginger Compress for Muscle Soreness

- Simmer grated ginger in hot water for 10 minutes. Soak a cloth in the liquid, wring it out, and place it on sore areas.

14. Turmeric Golden Milk for Muscle Recovery

- Warm 1 cup milk (dairy or plant-based) with 1/2 teaspoon turmeric powder and a pinch of black pepper.
- Sweeten with honey and drink to reduce muscle

inflammation.

15. **Cayenne Salve for Muscle Pain**

- Melt 1/4 cup coconut oil with 1 tablespoon beeswax, then stir in 1 teaspoon cayenne powder.
- Cool and apply sparingly to sore muscles. (Test on a small area first.)

16. **Basil and Lavender Massage Oil**

- Mix 10 drops lavender oil and 5 drops basil oil into 1/4 cup carrier oil.
- Use for gentle massage to ease muscle tightness.

17. **Devil's Claw Tea for Chronic Pain**

- Steep 1 teaspoon dried devil's claw root in boiling water for 15 minutes.
- Drink 1–2 cups daily for muscle and joint pain relief.

18. **Peppermint Muscle Spray**

- Combine 1/4 cup witch hazel with 10 drops peppermint essential oil in a spray bottle.
- Spray onto sore muscles for cooling relief.

19. **Comfrey and Arnica Poultice for Pain Relief**

- Mix dried comfrey and arnica flowers with a little warm water to form a paste.
- Apply to sore areas, cover with a cloth, and leave for 15 minutes.

20. **Magnesium-Rich Nettle and Oat Straw Tea**

- Brew equal parts nettle and oat straw in hot water for 15 minutes.
- Drink daily to relax muscles and reduce soreness.

Remedies for Joint Pain

21. Ginger and Turmeric Joint Tea

- Simmer 1 teaspoon grated ginger and 1/2 teaspoon turmeric in 2 cups water for 10 minutes.
- Drink twice daily to reduce inflammation and ease arthritis pain.

22. Dandelion Leaf and Root Tea for Joint Health

- Steep 1 teaspoon each of dandelion root and leaves in boiling water for 10 minutes.
- Drink daily to reduce joint swelling and detoxify the body.

23. White Willow Bark and Devil's Claw Joint Tonic

- Combine equal parts of white willow bark and devil's claw in a tea blend.
- Steep 1 teaspoon in hot water for 15 minutes and drink daily.

24. St. John's Wort Massage Oil

- Infuse St. John's Wort flowers in olive oil for 4 weeks, then strain.
- Massage onto stiff joints to reduce pain and inflammation.

25. Rosemary and Cayenne Joint Rub

- Mix 1 tablespoon cayenne powder with 1/4 cup rosemary-infused oil.
- Massage onto joints for warming pain relief.

26. Nettle and Horsetail Joint Tea

- Brew 1 teaspoon each of dried nettle and horsetail in boiling water.
- Drink daily to provide minerals that support joint health.

27. Bone Broth Infused with Anti-Inflammatory Spices

- Simmer bone broth with ginger, turmeric, and garlic.
- Drink daily to nourish joints and reduce pain.

28. Calendula and Chamomile Compress

- Steep equal parts calendula and chamomile flowers in hot water, soak a cloth, and apply to swollen joints.

29. Burdock Root Tea for Joint Detox

- Simmer 1 teaspoon dried burdock root in 2 cups water for 15 minutes.
- Drink daily to reduce inflammation and cleanse the blood.

30. Epsom Salt and Lavender Compress

- Dissolve 1/2 cup Epsom salts in warm water, soak a cloth, and apply to achy joints for 20 minutes.

2.4 IMMUNE BOOSTERS AND SEASONAL ILLNESSES

When seasonal illnesses like fevers, flu, and fatigue hit, herbal remedies can provide gentle yet powerful support to help the body recover. This chapter provides 30 remedies to boost the immune system, manage fever, soothe flu symptoms, and combat fatigue during and after illness. These time-tested solutions combine herbs with antiviral, adaptogenic, and immune-enhancing properties to ease symptoms and promote recovery.

Remedies for Fevers

1. Elderflower and Peppermint Fever Tea

- Combine 1 teaspoon each of dried elderflowers and peppermint leaves in 1 cup boiling water.
- Steep for 10 minutes, strain, and drink to encourage sweating and lower fever.

2. Ginger and Cinnamon Fever Reducer

- Simmer 1 teaspoon grated ginger and 1 cinnamon stick in 2 cups water for 10 minutes.
- Drink warm to stimulate circulation and reduce chills.

3. Apple Cider Vinegar Compress for Fevers

- Mix 1/4 cup apple cider vinegar with 1/4 cup cool water.
- Soak a cloth in the mixture and place it on the forehead or wrists to cool the body naturally.

4. Yarrow Tea for Fever Management

- Steep 1 teaspoon dried yarrow in 1 cup boiling water for 10 minutes.
- Drink to promote sweating and help the body break a fever.

5. Lemon Balm Fever Relief Tea

- Brew 1 teaspoon dried lemon balm in 1 cup boiling water.
- Drink 2–3 times daily to relax the body and reduce fever.

6. Peppermint and Chamomile Cooling Tea

- Combine 1 teaspoon each of peppermint and chamomile in hot water.
- Drink to calm the body, reduce fever, and soothe inflammation.

7. Raw Onion Fever Compress

- Slice a raw onion and place the slices on the bottoms of your feet.
- Secure with socks and leave overnight to help draw heat from the body.

8. Ginger Foot Bath

- Add 2 tablespoons grated fresh ginger to a basin of warm water.

- Soak your feet for 15–20 minutes to improve circulation and reduce fever.

9. White Willow Bark Decoction

- Simmer 1 teaspoon white willow bark in 2 cups water for 15 minutes.
- Drink to reduce fever and relieve aches. (White willow bark contains salicin, similar to aspirin.)

10. Basil Fever Remedy

- Steep 1 teaspoon dried basil leaves in hot water.
- Drink warm to lower fever and support respiratory health.

Remedies for Flu

11. Elderberry and Ginger Flu Tea

- Simmer 1/4 cup dried elderberries with 1 tablespoon grated ginger in 3 cups water for 20 minutes.
- Strain, sweeten with honey, and sip to boost immunity and reduce flu symptoms.

12. Garlic and Honey Flu Remedy

- Crush 2–3 garlic cloves and mix with 1/4 cup raw honey.
- Take 1 teaspoon every few hours to fight infection and soothe a sore throat.

13. Thyme Steam Inhalation

- Add 1 tablespoon dried thyme to a bowl of steaming water.
- Inhale deeply to clear sinuses and reduce congestion.

14. Chamomile and Lavender Flu Bath

- Add 1/4 cup dried chamomile and 1/4 cup dried lavender to a hot bath.
- Soak to relax sore muscles and relieve flu-related aches.

15. Cinnamon and Clove Antiviral Tea

- Simmer 1 cinnamon stick and 2 cloves in 2 cups water for 10 minutes.
- Drink to reduce inflammation and fight flu viruses.

16. Reishi Mushroom Immune Support Tonic

- Simmer 1 tablespoon dried reishi mushroom in 3 cups water for 30 minutes.
- Sip to strengthen the immune system and reduce flu severity.

17. Pine Needle Flu Tea

- Steep fresh pine needles in hot water for 10 minutes.
- Drink to clear lungs, detoxify the body, and boost vitamin C levels.

18. Eucalyptus and Peppermint Chest Rub

- Mix 1/4 cup coconut oil with 10 drops eucalyptus essential oil and 5 drops peppermint oil.
- Massage onto the chest to ease breathing and reduce congestion.

19. Elderberry and Rosehip Vitamin C Tea

- Combine 1 teaspoon each of dried elderberries and rosehips in hot water.

- Steep for 10 minutes and drink to boost immunity and speed recovery.

20. Oregano Oil Steam for Flu Symptoms

- Add 2 drops oregano essential oil to a bowl of hot water.
- Inhale deeply to relieve respiratory symptoms and support recovery.

Remedies for Fatigue During and After Illness

21. Ashwagandha Energy Tonic

- Mix 1 teaspoon ashwagandha powder into warm almond milk.
- Add honey and drink daily to restore energy and fight post-illness fatigue.

22. Adaptogenic Chai Latte

- Brew chai tea with 1 teaspoon each of ashwagandha and reishi mushroom powders.
- Add milk and honey for a warming, energizing drink.

23. Holy Basil (Tulsi) and Ginger Revitalizing Tea

- Steep 1 teaspoon dried holy basil and 1 teaspoon grated ginger in hot water.
- Drink to reduce stress and combat fatigue.

24. Nettle and Oat Straw Mineral Infusion

- Steep 1 tablespoon each of dried nettle and oat straw in 1 quart boiling water for 4–8 hours.

- Drink throughout the day to nourish the body and restore energy.

25. Licorice Root and Cinnamon Energy Tea

- Simmer 1 teaspoon dried licorice root and 1 cinnamon stick in 2 cups water.
- Sip to combat adrenal fatigue and boost energy.

26. Bone Broth Recovery Drink

- Simmer bone broth with garlic, turmeric, and ginger.
- Sip throughout the day to nourish the body and promote healing.

27. Lemon Balm and Lavender Stress Relief Tea

- Brew 1 teaspoon dried lemon balm with 1/2 teaspoon lavender in hot water.
- Drink to calm the nervous system and reduce post-illness fatigue.

28. Honey and Ginseng Tonic

- Mix 1 teaspoon honey with 1/4 teaspoon powdered ginseng in warm water.
- Drink daily to restore vitality and fight fatigue.

29. Adaptogenic Smoothie

- Blend 1 teaspoon ashwagandha powder, 1 tablespoon chia seeds, 1 banana, and 1 cup almond milk.
- Drink as a nourishing energy booster.

30. Golden Milk Recovery Drink

- Combine 1 teaspoon turmeric powder, a pinch of black pepper, and 1/4 teaspoon cinnamon in warm milk.
- Sweeten with honey and sip to reduce inflammation and restore energy.

PART 3: HOLISTIC BEAUTY AND SELF-CARE

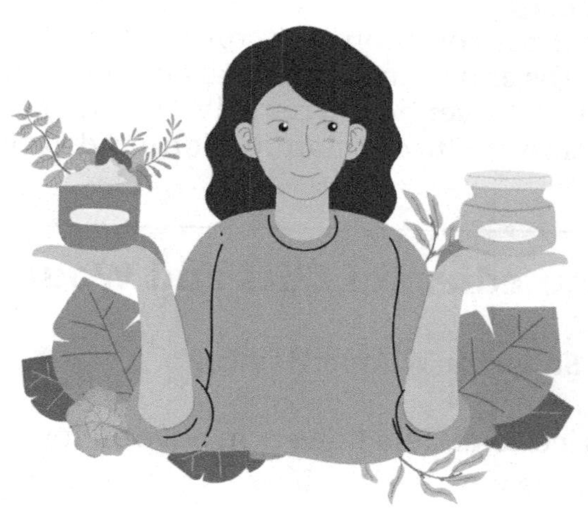

3.1 SKIN HEALING REMEDIES

Your skin is your body's largest organ and your first line of defense against the outside world. Cuts, burns, rashes, and acne are common skin concerns, but nature provides a wealth of herbs and remedies to heal and nourish your skin. In this chapter, we'll cover herbal remedies to support skin healing, soothe irritation, reduce inflammation, and promote natural radiance.

Remedies for Cuts and Wounds

1. Calendula Salve for Wound Healing

- Infuse dried calendula flowers in olive oil for 4 weeks, strain, and combine with melted beeswax to make a salve.
- Apply to cuts and scrapes to reduce inflammation and promote healing.

2. Honey Wound Dressing

- Apply a thin layer of raw honey directly to a clean wound.
- Cover with a sterile bandage to prevent infection and speed healing.

3. Yarrow Poultice for Bleeding

- Crush fresh yarrow leaves into a paste and apply directly to a bleeding wound.

- Yarrow is a natural styptic and helps stop bleeding while reducing infection risk.

4. Lavender and Tea Tree Antiseptic Spray

- Combine 1/4 cup witch hazel with 10 drops lavender oil and 5 drops tea tree oil in a spray bottle.
- Spray onto cuts to cleanse and disinfect.

5. Plantain Poultice for Minor Cuts

- Mash fresh plantain leaves and apply them to cuts and scrapes.
- Cover with a bandage to soothe inflammation and promote healing.

6. Comfrey Healing Compress

- Steep 1 tablespoon dried comfrey leaves in hot water for 10 minutes.
- Soak a cloth in the tea and apply it to wounds to promote tissue repair.

7. Aloe Vera Gel for Minor Cuts

- Apply fresh aloe vera gel directly to small cuts to soothe and speed healing.

8. Chamomile Wash for Wounds

- Brew a strong chamomile tea and let it cool. Use as a gentle antiseptic wash for cuts and scrapes.

9. Goldenseal and Myrrh Powder Dusting

- Mix equal parts goldenseal and myrrh powder. Sprinkle over a wound to keep it clean and aid healing.

10. Garlic and Honey Infection Fighter

- Mix crushed garlic with raw honey and apply to infected wounds.
- Cover with a bandage to reduce bacteria and inflammation.

Remedies for Burns

11. Aloe Vera Gel for Burns

- Apply fresh aloe vera gel directly to minor burns to cool the skin and promote healing.

12. Lavender Burn Spray

- Mix 1/4 cup distilled water with 10 drops lavender essential oil in a spray bottle.
- Spray onto minor burns to reduce pain and inflammation.

13. St. John's Wort Oil for Sunburn

- Apply St. John's Wort-infused oil to sunburned skin for quick relief and healing.

14. Raw Honey Burn Dressing

- Spread a thin layer of raw honey onto a sterile gauze pad and apply it to minor burns.
- Honey is cooling and antimicrobial, helping to prevent infection.

15. Calendula and Chamomile Burn Soak

- Brew a strong tea with equal parts calendula and

chamomile.

- Let it cool, then soak a clean cloth in the tea and apply to burned areas.

16. Peppermint and Aloe Cooling Gel

- Mix fresh aloe vera gel with a few drops of peppermint essential oil.
- Apply to burns to cool the skin and reduce redness.

17. Plantain Infusion for Burn Relief

- Brew a strong tea with fresh or dried plantain leaves and let it cool.
- Use as a compress to soothe burns and reduce inflammation.

18. Vitamin E Oil for Burn Healing

- Break open a vitamin E capsule and apply the oil directly to burns.
- This helps reduce scarring and promote skin repair.

19. Marshmallow Root Burn Wash

- Simmer 1 tablespoon dried marshmallow root in 2 cups water for 15 minutes.
- Strain and use the cooled tea as a soothing wash for burns.

20. Turmeric and Honey Burn Paste

- Mix 1 teaspoon turmeric powder with 1 tablespoon honey to form a paste.
- Apply to burns to reduce inflammation and prevent

infection.

Remedies for Rashes and Skin Irritation

21. Oatmeal Bath for Itchy Rashes

- Grind 1 cup oats into a fine powder and add it to a warm bath.
- Soak for 15–20 minutes to soothe irritated, itchy skin.

22. Calendula and Plantain Rash Cream

- Infuse calendula and plantain in olive oil, strain, and mix with melted beeswax.
- Apply to rashes to calm irritation and reduce redness.

23. Witch Hazel Compress for Rashes

- Soak a cloth in witch hazel and apply it to irritated skin to reduce inflammation and itching.

24. Chamomile and Lavender Anti-Itch Spray

- Combine 1/4 cup witch hazel with 10 drops chamomile essential oil and 10 drops lavender oil in a spray bottle.
- Spray onto rashes or insect bites for soothing relief.

25. Nettle Leaf Tea for Eczema

- Brew 1 tablespoon dried nettle in 2 cups boiling water for 10 minutes.
- Drink daily to reduce inflammation and support skin health.

26. Peppermint and Cucumber Soothing Paste

- Blend fresh peppermint leaves with cucumber slices to form a paste.
- Apply to rashes to cool the skin and reduce redness.

27. Goldenseal and Calendula Anti-Rash Salve

- Mix goldenseal powder with calendula-infused oil and beeswax to create a salve.
- Apply to rashes to speed healing and fight infection.

28. Coconut Oil with Tea Tree for Fungal Rashes

- Mix 1 tablespoon coconut oil with 5 drops tea tree essential oil.
- Apply to areas affected by fungal rashes.

29. Chickweed Poultice for Poison Ivy

- Mash fresh chickweed leaves and apply directly to the rash.
- Cover with a bandage to soothe itching and irritation.

30. Epsom Salt and Lavender Soak for Rashes

- Dissolve 1 cup Epsom salts and 10 drops lavender essential oil in a warm bath.
- Soak to reduce inflammation and calm itchy skin.

3.2 EVERYDAY SKINCARE

Herbs are nature's gift to our skin, offering gentle, effective solutions to cleanse, hydrate, tone, and nourish. This chapter focuses on herbal remedies to create simple, luxurious masks, toners, and moisturizers that promote radiant and healthy skin. Whether you're looking to brighten dull skin, balance oiliness, or deeply hydrate, these remedies will help you build a natural skincare routine that works.

Herbal Masks for Cleansing and Nourishment

1. Oatmeal and Chamomile Soothing Mask

- Blend 2 tablespoons finely ground oats with 2 tablespoons chamomile tea.
- Apply to your face and let sit for 15 minutes.
- Perfect for calming irritated or sensitive skin.

2. Honey and Turmeric Brightening Mask

- Mix 1 tablespoon raw honey with 1/2 teaspoon turmeric powder.
- Apply to your face for 10–15 minutes, then rinse.
- Helps reduce inflammation and brighten skin tone.

3. Bentonite Clay and Peppermint Oil Detox Mask

- Combine 1 tablespoon bentonite clay with enough water to

form a paste.

- Add 1–2 drops peppermint essential oil. Apply to your face and let dry before rinsing.
- Ideal for oily or acne-prone skin.

4. Aloe Vera and Cucumber Hydrating Mask

- Blend 2 tablespoons fresh aloe vera gel with 2 tablespoons cucumber juice.
- Apply to your face and let sit for 15 minutes to refresh and hydrate.

5. Matcha Green Tea Antioxidant Mask

- Mix 1 teaspoon matcha powder with 1 tablespoon yogurt.
- Apply to your face and leave on for 15 minutes to fight free radicals and reduce redness.

6. Avocado and Honey Moisturizing Mask

- Mash 1/4 ripe avocado and mix with 1 tablespoon honey.
- Apply to your face for deep hydration and nourishment.

7. Rose Petal and Yogurt Glow Mask

- Blend 2 tablespoons fresh rose petals with 1 tablespoon plain yogurt.
- Apply to your face to soften and brighten your complexion.

8. Activated Charcoal and Tea Tree Detox Mask

- Mix 1 teaspoon activated charcoal powder with 1 tablespoon water and 2 drops tea tree oil.

- Apply to draw out impurities and reduce acne.

9. Carrot and Honey Revitalizing Mask

- Mix 1 tablespoon carrot juice with 1 tablespoon honey.
- Apply to brighten tired, dull skin.

10. Calendula and Coconut Oil Soothing Mask

- Blend dried calendula petals into a powder and mix with 1 tablespoon coconut oil.
- Apply to soothe inflamed or irritated skin.

Herbal Toners for Refreshing and Balancing Skin

11. Rosewater Toner

- Fill a spray bottle with pure rosewater.
- Use as a toner to hydrate and balance skin after cleansing.

12. Green Tea Antioxidant Toner

- Brew 1 cup green tea and let it cool.
- Store in a spray bottle and use to tone and refresh skin throughout the day.

13. Witch Hazel and Lavender Toner

- Combine 1/4 cup witch hazel with 5 drops lavender essential oil.
- Apply with a cotton pad to balance oil and soothe skin.

14. Cucumber and Mint Cooling Toner

- Blend cucumber juice with a handful of fresh mint leaves.
- Strain and store in the fridge. Apply to calm redness and cool the skin.

15. Chamomile and Aloe Vera Toner

- Steep 1 tablespoon chamomile flowers in 1 cup boiling water. Let cool and mix with 2 tablespoons aloe vera gel.
- Use to hydrate sensitive skin.

16. Apple Cider Vinegar Balancing Toner

- Mix 1 part apple cider vinegar with 2 parts distilled water.
- Apply to the face with a cotton pad to balance pH and reduce oiliness.

17. Hibiscus and Rose Toner

- Steep 1 tablespoon dried hibiscus flowers with rose petals in hot water for 10 minutes.
- Let cool and apply to brighten and refresh skin.

18. Witch Hazel and Tea Tree Oil Acne Toner

- Combine 1/4 cup witch hazel with 5 drops tea tree oil.
- Apply to blemish-prone areas to reduce acne and inflammation.

19. Lemon Balm and Peppermint Energizing Toner

- Brew equal parts lemon balm and peppermint tea.
- Let cool and store in the fridge for a refreshing morning toner.

20. Nettle and Lavender Toner for Oily Skin

- Brew 1 tablespoon dried nettle with lavender flowers in 1 cup hot water.
- Cool and use to balance oily skin and reduce redness.

Herbal Moisturizers for Deep Hydration

21. Aloe Vera and Jojoba Oil Lightweight Moisturizer

- Mix 2 tablespoons aloe vera gel with 1 tablespoon jojoba oil.
- Apply as a lightweight, non-greasy moisturizer for all skin types.

22. Calendula and Shea Butter Balm

- Infuse calendula petals in olive oil, then mix with melted shea butter and beeswax.
- Use as a rich moisturizer for dry or irritated skin.

23. Coconut Oil and Lavender Night Cream

- Mix 1/4 cup coconut oil with 10 drops lavender essential oil.
- Apply before bed to hydrate and relax your skin.

24. Rosehip and Argan Oil Anti-Aging Serum

- Combine 2 tablespoons rosehip oil with 1 tablespoon argan oil.
- Massage into your skin to reduce fine lines and improve elasticity.

25. Aloe and Vitamin E Hydrating Gel

- Mix 2 tablespoons aloe vera gel with the oil from 1 vitamin E capsule.
- Use for deep hydration and to soothe dry patches.

26. Chamomile-Infused Olive Oil for Dry Skin

- Infuse chamomile flowers in olive oil for 4 weeks.
- Apply to dry skin for nourishment and calming.

27. Cucumber and Honey Gel Moisturizer

- Blend fresh cucumber with 1 tablespoon honey and strain to make a lightweight gel.
- Apply to your face for a refreshing boost of hydration.

28. Nettle and Oat Hydrating Cream

- Infuse nettle leaves in water and mix with colloidal oats and a small amount of shea butter.
- Apply to soothe dryness and nourish the skin barrier.

29. Lavender and Beeswax Face Balm

- Melt 1/4 cup beeswax with 1/4 cup almond oil and add 5 drops lavender oil.
- Let cool and use as a rich, protective moisturizer for dry or cold-weather skin.

30. Aloe and Calendula Oil Face Cream

- Mix aloe vera gel with calendula-infused oil and a small amount of shea butter.
- Apply as a daily moisturizer for glowing skin.

3.3 HAIR CARE REMEDIES

Your hair is a reflection of your overall health, and herbs can help you nurture it from root to tip. Whether you're dealing with a dry, flaky scalp, thinning hair, or dull strands, herbal remedies can stimulate growth, improve scalp health, and add natural shine. This chapter offers remedies for nourishing your hair with scalp treatments, growth oils, and shine-boosting rinses.

Scalp Treatments for Health and Balance

1. Rosemary and Tea Tree Scalp Oil

- Combine 2 tablespoons coconut oil with 5 drops rosemary oil and 3 drops tea tree oil.
- Massage into the scalp to improve circulation and fight dandruff.

2. Nettle and Horsetail Scalp Rinse

- Brew 1 tablespoon each of nettle and horsetail in 2 cups boiling water.
- Let cool, strain, and use as a final rinse to strengthen the scalp and promote hair growth.

3. Aloe Vera and Lavender Scalp Soothing Mask

- Mix 2 tablespoons fresh aloe vera gel with 3 drops lavender essential oil.

- Apply to the scalp to soothe irritation and hydrate dry skin.

4. **Apple Cider Vinegar Clarifying Rinse**

    - Mix 1/4 cup apple cider vinegar with 2 cups water.
    - Pour over your scalp after shampooing to remove buildup and restore pH balance.

5. **Fenugreek and Lemon Anti-Dandruff Treatment**

    - Soak 2 tablespoons fenugreek seeds overnight and blend into a paste.
    - Mix with 1 tablespoon lemon juice and apply to the scalp for 30 minutes before rinsing.

6. **Chamomile and Calendula Calming Scalp Rinse**

    - Brew 1 tablespoon each of chamomile and calendula in 2 cups water.
    - Strain and pour over your scalp to reduce redness and irritation.

7. **Peppermint and Eucalyptus Cooling Scalp Mist**

    - Combine 1/4 cup distilled water with 3 drops peppermint oil and 3 drops eucalyptus oil.
    - Spray onto the scalp for a refreshing, cooling treatment.

8. **Neem Oil Anti-Fungal Scalp Treatment**

    - Mix 1 tablespoon neem oil with 2 tablespoons olive oil.
    - Massage into the scalp to fight dandruff and fungal infections.

9. **Baking Soda and Tea Tree Exfoliating Scrub**

- Mix 1 tablespoon baking soda with a few drops tea tree oil and enough water to make a paste.
- Gently scrub the scalp to remove flakes and buildup.

10. Oat Milk and Honey Scalp Mask

- Blend 1/4 cup oat milk with 1 tablespoon honey.
- Massage into the scalp to soothe dryness and nourish skin.

Herbal Growth Oils for Stronger, Thicker Hair

11. Rosemary and Castor Hair Growth Oil

- Combine 1/4 cup castor oil with 10 drops rosemary essential oil.
- Massage into your scalp and leave overnight to stimulate hair growth.

12. Onion Juice and Aloe Growth Treatment

- Blend 1/4 cup fresh onion juice with 2 tablespoons aloe vera gel.
- Apply to the scalp to boost circulation and promote growth.

13. Horsetail and Olive Oil Strengthening Serum

- Infuse 2 tablespoons dried horsetail in 1/4 cup olive oil for 2 weeks, then strain.
- Massage into the scalp to strengthen hair roots.

14. Fenugreek and Coconut Growth Oil

- Heat 2 tablespoons coconut oil with 1 teaspoon fenugreek

seeds.

- Let cool and apply to the scalp to improve thickness and reduce shedding.

15. Garlic and Mustard Seed Hair Growth Oil

- Heat 1/4 cup mustard seed oil with 2 crushed garlic cloves.
- Strain and massage into the scalp to promote growth.

16. Amla and Sesame Hair Growth Oil

- Mix 1/4 cup sesame oil with 1 tablespoon powdered amla (Indian gooseberry).
- Massage into the scalp and leave on for 1 hour before rinsing.

17. Lavender and Argan Oil Restorative Serum

- Mix 2 tablespoons argan oil with 5 drops lavender essential oil.
- Apply to the scalp to reduce stress and improve hair growth.

18. Black Seed Oil Hair Growth Treatment

- Massage 1–2 tablespoons black seed oil into your scalp and hair roots.
- Leave on overnight for stronger, healthier hair.

19. Basil and Castor Oil Infusion

- Infuse 2 tablespoons dried basil in 1/4 cup castor oil for 2 weeks.
- Strain and apply to the scalp to encourage growth.

20. Ginger and Jojoba Hair Oil

- Grate 1 tablespoon fresh ginger and mix with 2 tablespoons jojoba oil.
- Massage into the scalp to improve circulation and promote hair growth.

Herbal Rinses and Shine Boosters

21. Rosemary and Sage Shine Rinse

- Brew 1 tablespoon each of rosemary and sage in 2 cups boiling water.
- Strain and pour over hair as a final rinse to add shine and darken graying hair.

22. Hibiscus and Rose Shine Rinse

- Steep 1 tablespoon dried hibiscus flowers and 1 tablespoon dried rose petals in 2 cups hot water.
- Strain and use as a final rinse to add softness and shine.

23. Green Tea and Lemon Shine Booster

- Brew 2 cups green tea and mix with the juice of 1 lemon.
- Pour over hair after washing to boost shine and cleanse the scalp.

24. Apple Cider Vinegar and Rosemary Rinse

- Combine 1/4 cup apple cider vinegar with 1 cup rosemary tea.
- Use as a final rinse to enhance shine and reduce frizz.

25. Chamomile and Lemon Rinse for Blonde Hair

- Brew 2 tablespoons dried chamomile in 2 cups boiling water. Add 1 tablespoon lemon juice.
- Pour over blonde hair to enhance highlights and add shine.

26. Black Tea Rinse for Dark Hair

- Brew a strong black tea and let it cool.
- Pour over dark hair to enhance richness and reduce dullness.

27. Calendula and Aloe Shine Mist

- Brew 1 tablespoon calendula flowers in 1 cup hot water. Let cool, strain, and mix with 1 tablespoon aloe vera gel.
- Spray onto hair to add shine and moisture.

28. Coconut Milk Shine Conditioner

- Massage 1/4 cup coconut milk into your hair after washing.
- Rinse out after 5–10 minutes for silky, shiny locks.

29. Lavender and Honey Hydrating Rinse

- Mix 1 tablespoon honey with 2 cups lavender tea.
- Pour over hair to lock in moisture and add a natural shine.

30. Peppermint and Nettle Strengthening Rinse

- Brew 1 tablespoon each of peppermint and nettle in 2 cups boiling water.
- Use as a final rinse to strengthen hair and add a healthy shine.

3.4 ANTI-AGING AND RADIANCE

Aging is a natural process, but we can use herbal remedies to nurture and restore the skin, promoting vitality and radiance. Herbs are rich in antioxidants, vitamins, and compounds that boost collagen, improve elasticity, and reduce the appearance of wrinkles. In this chapter, we'll explore remedies to rejuvenate your skin, soften fine lines, and enhance your glow.

Herbal Masks for Radiance and Wrinkle Reduction

1. Aloe Vera and Rosehip Anti-Wrinkle Mask

- Mix 2 tablespoons fresh aloe vera gel with 1 teaspoon rosehip seed oil.
- Apply to your face for 20 minutes to hydrate and boost collagen production.

2. Green Tea and Honey Brightening Mask

- Brew 1 teaspoon green tea and mix with 1 tablespoon honey.
- Apply to your face for 15 minutes to fight free radicals and brighten skin.

3. Turmeric and Yogurt Collagen Mask

- Mix 1 tablespoon plain yogurt with 1/2 teaspoon turmeric powder.
- Apply to your face to tighten skin and reduce inflammation.

4. **Avocado and Vitamin E Nourishing Mask**
   - Mash 1/4 avocado with the oil from a vitamin E capsule.
   - Apply to your face for deep hydration and wrinkle reduction.
5. **Hibiscus and Oat Hydrating Mask**
   - Blend 1 teaspoon ground hibiscus flowers with 2 tablespoons oatmeal and enough water to form a paste.
   - Apply to plump and hydrate dry skin.
6. **Cucumber and Aloe Cooling Mask**
   - Blend fresh cucumber with aloe vera gel and apply to your face.
   - Reduces puffiness and refreshes tired skin.
7. **Banana and Honey Wrinkle-Repair Mask**
   - Mash 1/2 ripe banana and mix with 1 tablespoon honey.
   - Apply to soften fine lines and moisturize the skin.
8. **Carrot and Honey Revitalizing Mask**
   - Blend 2 tablespoons carrot juice with 1 tablespoon honey.
   - Apply to your face for a radiant glow and reduced wrinkles.
9. **Rose Petal and Milk Anti-Aging Mask**

- Blend fresh rose petals with 2 tablespoons milk.
- Apply for soft, glowing skin.

10. Papaya and Green Tea Enzyme Mask

- Mash 2 tablespoons papaya and mix with 1 teaspoon brewed green tea.
- Apply to exfoliate and renew skin cells.

Herbal Toners to Firm and Refresh Skin

11. Witch Hazel and Rosewater Toner

- Mix 1/4 cup witch hazel with 1/4 cup rosewater.
- Apply with a cotton pad to firm and hydrate skin after cleansing.

12. Green Tea and Cucumber Toner

- Brew 1 cup green tea, let cool, and mix with 2 tablespoons cucumber juice.
- Use as a refreshing, antioxidant-rich toner to tighten pores.

13. Aloe Vera and Lemon Brightening Toner

- Mix 1/4 cup aloe vera gel with the juice of 1/2 lemon.
- Use to brighten dull skin and reduce dark spots.

14. Chamomile and Lavender Hydrating Toner

- Brew 1 tablespoon dried chamomile flowers with 1 tablespoon dried lavender in 1 cup hot water.
- Strain and use to hydrate and calm irritated skin.

15. Hibiscus and Rose Antioxidant Toner

- Brew 1 tablespoon each of hibiscus and dried rose petals in hot water.
- Strain and store in a spray bottle for a vitamin C-rich toner.

16. Apple Cider Vinegar and Green Tea pH Balancing Toner

- Mix 1/4 cup apple cider vinegar with 1/4 cup green tea.
- Apply to balance skin's pH and promote smoothness.

17. Basil and Mint Pore-Refining Toner

- Brew 1 tablespoon each of basil and mint in 1 cup hot water.
- Use to reduce oiliness and minimize pores.

18. Lemon Balm and Peppermint Refreshing Toner

- Brew equal parts lemon balm and peppermint in 1 cup hot water.
- Use to energize and refresh skin.

19. Cucumber and Witch Hazel Firming Mist

- Blend 1/4 cup cucumber juice with 1/4 cup witch hazel.
- Spray onto your face to firm and hydrate throughout the day.

20. Lavender and Honey Hydrating Mist

- Brew 1 tablespoon dried lavender in hot water and mix with 1 teaspoon honey.
- Use as a hydrating mist to reduce dryness.

Herbal Oils and Serums for Wrinkle Reduction

21. Rosehip and Argan Oil Serum

- Combine 2 tablespoons rosehip seed oil with 1 tablespoon argan oil.
- Massage onto your face to improve elasticity and reduce wrinkles.

22. Pomegranate and Jojoba Repair Serum

- Mix 2 tablespoons jojoba oil with 1 tablespoon pomegranate seed oil.
- Apply at night to reduce fine lines and promote cell regeneration.

23. Calendula-Infused Olive Oil

- Infuse dried calendula flowers in olive oil for 2–4 weeks.
- Strain and massage onto skin to hydrate and calm inflammation.

24. Aloe Vera and Vitamin E Repair Gel

- Mix 2 tablespoons aloe vera gel with the oil from 2 vitamin E capsules.
- Apply to repair damaged skin and boost collagen.

25. Green Tea and Grapeseed Oil Serum

- Mix 2 tablespoons grapeseed oil with 1 teaspoon brewed green tea.
- Use to fight free radicals and tighten skin.

26. Lavender and Carrot Seed Night Oil

- Mix 2 tablespoons almond oil with 5 drops lavender oil and 3 drops carrot seed oil.
- Apply before bed for skin renewal.

27. Sea Buckthorn and Argan Oil Glow Serum

- Combine 1 tablespoon sea buckthorn oil with 1 tablespoon argan oil.
- Massage into skin to promote radiance and reduce dryness.

28. Frankincense and Jojoba Anti-Aging Serum

- Mix 2 tablespoons jojoba oil with 5 drops frankincense essential oil.
- Apply to reduce wrinkles and promote skin firmness.

29. Coconut and Geranium Restorative Oil

- Combine 2 tablespoons coconut oil with 5 drops geranium essential oil.
- Apply to hydrate and tone skin.

30. Turmeric and Almond Oil Glow Serum

- Mix 1 tablespoon almond oil with 1/4 teaspoon turmeric powder.
- Massage into your skin for a radiant, youthful glow.

PART 4: EMOTIONAL AND MENTAL WELLNESS

4.1 RELAXATION AND STRESS RELIEF

In today's fast-paced world, stress and tension can take a toll on both body and mind. Herbs offer gentle, effective ways to relax, reduce anxiety, and promote a sense of calm. This chapter includes remedies—a mix of calming teas, soothing tinctures, and aromatic blends to help you unwind and restore balance.

Calming Teas for Relaxation

1. Chamomile and Lavender Bedtime Tea

- Steep 1 teaspoon dried chamomile flowers and 1/2 teaspoon dried lavender in 1 cup boiling water for 10 minutes.
- Drink before bed to relax your mind and promote restful sleep.

2. Lemon Balm Relaxation Tea

- Brew 1 tablespoon dried lemon balm leaves in 1 cup boiling water for 10 minutes.
- Drink to ease nervousness and promote calm.

3. Peppermint and Rose Petal Stress-Soothing Tea

- Combine 1 teaspoon dried peppermint leaves with 1 teaspoon dried rose petals.

- Brew for 10 minutes to soothe tension and uplift your mood.

4. Passionflower Anxiety Tea

- Steep 1 teaspoon dried passionflower in 1 cup boiling water for 10 minutes.
- Drink during moments of high stress to calm racing thoughts.

5. Holy Basil (Tulsi) Adaptogenic Tea

- Brew 1 teaspoon dried tulsi in hot water for 10 minutes.
- Drink daily to support your body's response to stress.

6. Oat Straw and Chamomile Nervine Tea

- Combine 1 tablespoon oat straw with 1 teaspoon chamomile in boiling water.
- Sip to nourish the nervous system and promote relaxation.

7. Valerian Root and Lemon Balm Sleep Tea

- Simmer 1 teaspoon valerian root in 1 cup water for 5 minutes.
- Add 1 teaspoon lemon balm and steep for another 10 minutes.
- Drink before bed for deep, restorative sleep.

8. Rose and Hibiscus Heart-Opening Tea

- Steep 1 teaspoon dried rose petals and 1 teaspoon hibiscus flowers in 1 cup hot water.
- Drink to calm the heart and promote emotional balance.

9. Peppermint and Licorice Root Digestive Calm Tea

- Brew 1 teaspoon dried peppermint and 1/2 teaspoon dried licorice root.
- Drink to soothe digestion and calm stress-related upset stomachs.

10. Lavender and Lemon Zest Evening Tea

- Combine 1/2 teaspoon dried lavender flowers with fresh lemon zest.
- Brew in hot water for a refreshing yet calming nighttime tea.

Soothing Tinctures for Stress and Anxiety

11. Ashwagandha Adaptogenic Tincture

- Take 1–2 droppers of ashwagandha tincture (available commercially or homemade) daily.
- Helps reduce cortisol levels and build long-term stress resilience.

12. Lemon Balm Calming Tincture

- Steep fresh lemon balm leaves in vodka for 4–6 weeks.
- Take 1 dropper when you feel overwhelmed.

13. Passionflower Anti-Anxiety Tincture

- Use 1–2 droppers of passionflower tincture to relax the mind and reduce feelings of tension.

14. Holy Basil Stress-Reducing Tincture

- Infuse fresh tulsi leaves in alcohol for 4 weeks, strain, and take 1 dropper daily to balance mood and energy.

15. Valerian Root Sleep Aid Tincture

- Take 1 dropper of valerian root tincture 30 minutes before bed to promote restful sleep.

16. Skullcap Nervine Tincture

- Use 1–2 droppers of skullcap tincture when feeling overwhelmed or emotionally frazzled.

17. Lavender and Hops Relaxation Tincture

- Combine fresh lavender flowers and hops in vodka for 4 weeks, strain, and take 1 dropper before bedtime.

18. Chamomile and Lemon Balm Uplifting Tincture

- Mix dried chamomile and lemon balm in alcohol for 4–6 weeks.
- Take during the day for calm focus and reduced anxiety.

19. Milky Oat Stress Recovery Tincture

- Infuse fresh milky oat tops in vodka for 4 weeks.
- Take 1 dropper daily to repair and nourish an overworked nervous system.

20. Rose Petal Emotional Support Tincture

- Infuse fresh rose petals in alcohol for 4 weeks.
- Take 1–2 droppers to calm the heart and uplift the spirit.

Aromatherapy Blends for Relaxation

21. Lavender and Bergamot Diffuser Blend

- Add 4 drops lavender oil and 3 drops bergamot oil to a diffuser.
- Use to create a calm, peaceful atmosphere.

22. Peppermint and Eucalyptus Energy Reset Blend

- Combine 3 drops peppermint oil with 2 drops eucalyptus oil.
- Diffuse to clear the mind and boost mental clarity.

23. Frankincense and Sandalwood Grounding Blend

- Mix 4 drops frankincense oil with 3 drops sandalwood oil.
- Diffuse during meditation or quiet moments to promote grounding and relaxation.

24. Rose and Geranium Heart-Opening Blend

- Combine 3 drops rose oil and 3 drops geranium oil in a diffuser.
- Use to create a comforting and emotionally soothing environment.

25. Orange and Lavender Happy Blend

- Add 4 drops sweet orange oil and 2 drops lavender oil to a diffuser.
- Use during the day to uplift your mood and calm your nerves.

26. Ylang-Ylang and Lemon Calming Blend

- Mix 3 drops ylang-ylang oil with 3 drops lemon oil.
- Diffuse to create a calming, refreshing atmosphere.

27. Chamomile and Cedarwood Sleep Blend

- Add 4 drops chamomile oil and 3 drops cedarwood oil to a diffuser.
- Use before bedtime to promote deep relaxation.

28. Clary Sage and Rosemary Focus Blend

- Combine 3 drops clary sage oil and 2 drops rosemary oil.
- Diffuse to clear mental fog and ease tension headaches.

29. Patchouli and Lavender Stress Relief Blend

- Mix 3 drops patchouli oil with 3 drops lavender oil.
- Diffuse to ease stress and encourage a sense of balance.

30. Jasmine and Vanilla Comforting Blend

- Add 4 drops jasmine oil and 3 drops vanilla oil to a diffuser.
- Use for emotional soothing and to create a warm, calming atmosphere.

4.2 BETTER SLEEP SOLUTIONS

A good night's sleep is essential for physical health, mental clarity, and emotional well-being. Whether you're struggling with insomnia, restlessness, or racing thoughts, herbs can help you unwind and fall into a deep, restorative sleep. This chapter includes remedies—teas, tinctures, baths, and aromatherapy blends—that will naturally support your journey to peaceful slumber.

Calming Herbal Teas for Sleep

1. Chamomile and Lavender Sleep Tea

- Steep 1 teaspoon dried chamomile and 1/2 teaspoon dried lavender in 1 cup boiling water for 10 minutes.
- Drink 30 minutes before bed to calm the nervous system and promote relaxation.

2. Lemon Balm Sleep Tea

- Brew 1 tablespoon dried lemon balm in 1 cup boiling water for 10 minutes.
- Sip to reduce anxiety and quiet a racing mind.

3. Valerian Root Deep Sleep Tea

- Simmer 1 teaspoon dried valerian root in 2 cups water for 5–

10 minutes.

- Strain and drink to support deep and restorative sleep.

4. Passionflower Bedtime Tea

- Steep 1 teaspoon dried passionflower in 1 cup hot water for 10 minutes.

- Drink to calm overthinking and promote restful sleep.

5. Tulsi (Holy Basil) and Mint Tea

- Brew 1 teaspoon dried tulsi and 1 teaspoon dried peppermint in hot water for 10 minutes.

- Drink to calm the mind and soothe digestion before bed.

6. Lavender and Lemon Zest Tea

- Combine 1/2 teaspoon dried lavender flowers with fresh lemon zest in 1 cup boiling water.

- Drink to create a tranquil bedtime ritual.

7. Catnip Sleep Aid Tea

- Steep 1 teaspoon dried catnip in 1 cup hot water for 10 minutes.

- Catnip helps calm the nervous system and prepare the body for sleep.

8. Hops and Chamomile Sedative Tea

- Combine 1 teaspoon dried chamomile with 1/2 teaspoon dried hops flowers.

- Steep in boiling water for 10 minutes to support deep, uninterrupted sleep.

9. Oat Straw and Lemon Balm Tea

- Brew 1 tablespoon oat straw with 1 teaspoon lemon balm in hot water.
- Sip to nourish the nervous system and ease nighttime restlessness.

10. Rose and Hibiscus Sleep-Enhancing Tea

- Brew 1 teaspoon each of dried rose petals and hibiscus flowers.
- Drink to soothe emotions and calm the heart before bedtime.

Herbal Tinctures for Sleep Support

11. Valerian Root Sleep Tincture

- Take 1–2 droppers of valerian root tincture 30 minutes before bed to calm the mind and promote deep sleep.

12. Passionflower Anxiety-Reducing Tincture

- Use 1 dropper of passionflower tincture when your mind won't stop racing at bedtime.

13. Lavender and Skullcap Sleep Tincture

- Combine fresh lavender flowers and skullcap in alcohol for 4 weeks, strain, and take 1 dropper at bedtime to relax muscles and quiet the mind.

14. Hops Sedative Tincture

- Take 1 dropper of hops tincture before bed to encourage sleep and reduce anxiety.

15. Chamomile and Lemon Balm Calming Tincture

- Mix equal parts chamomile and lemon balm in vodka for 4 weeks.
- Take 1 dropper in the evening to wind down before bed.

16. Ashwagandha Adaptogenic Tincture

- Take 1–2 droppers of ashwagandha tincture daily to reduce cortisol levels and improve sleep quality over time.

17. California Poppy Sleep Tincture

- Use 1 dropper of California poppy tincture for a mild sedative effect to help you fall asleep faster.

18. Skullcap Nervous Tension Tincture

- Take 1 dropper of skullcap tincture to reduce restlessness and help ease into sleep.

19. Rose Petal and Holy Basil Emotional Support Tincture

- Take 1 dropper of this tincture to calm emotional tension and promote relaxation.

20. Milky Oat Tincture for Sleep Recovery

- Use 1 dropper of milky oat tincture to repair and nourish an overworked nervous system and improve sleep quality.

Herbal Baths for Restful Sleep

21. Lavender and Epsom Salt Bath

- Mix 1 cup Epsom salts with 10 drops lavender essential oil.
- Add to a warm bath and soak for 20 minutes to relax

muscles and calm the mind.

22. Chamomile and Rose Petal Bath Soak

- Brew a strong tea with 2 tablespoons dried chamomile and 2 tablespoons rose petals.
- Strain and add to your bath for a soothing, floral soak.

23. Hops and Oatmeal Sleep Bath

- Combine 1/4 cup dried hops flowers with 1/4 cup finely ground oats in a muslin bag.
- Drop into your bath to calm your body and mind.

24. Lemon Balm and Peppermint Relaxing Bath

- Brew a tea with 2 tablespoons dried lemon balm and 1 tablespoon dried peppermint.
- Add to your bath to ease tension and prepare for sleep.

25. Valerian Root Muscle-Relaxing Bath

- Simmer 1 tablespoon valerian root in 4 cups water for 10 minutes.
- Strain and add to your bath for a deep relaxation experience.

26. Calendula and Lavender Skin-Soothing Bath

- Brew a strong tea with 2 tablespoons calendula flowers and 2 tablespoons lavender flowers.
- Add to your bath for a calming soak that also soothes the skin.

27. Sandalwood and Chamomile Milk Bath

- Mix 1 cup milk with 1 teaspoon sandalwood powder and 2 tablespoons chamomile tea.
- Add to your bath to hydrate your skin and promote relaxation.

28. Magnesium-Rich Nettle and Epsom Salt Bath

- Brew 1/4 cup dried nettle in 4 cups water and add it to your bath with 1 cup Epsom salts.
- Soak to reduce muscle tension and improve sleep quality.

29. Frankincense and Cedarwood Grounding Bath

- Add 10 drops frankincense oil and 5 drops cedarwood oil to your bath.
- Soak to reduce anxiety and encourage a deep sense of calm.

30. Lavender and Peppermint Foot Soak

- Mix 1/4 cup Epsom salts with 5 drops lavender oil and 5 drops peppermint oil in warm water.
- Soak your feet for 15–20 minutes to relax your entire body.

4.3 MOOD AND FOCUS BOOSTERS

Your emotional and mental state impacts every aspect of your life, from productivity to relationships. Herbs can provide natural support for improving focus, uplifting your mood, and restoring mental clarity when you're feeling overwhelmed, distracted, or down. This chapter offers remedies—including teas, tinctures, aromatherapy blends, and tonics—to brighten your day, sharpen your mind, and help you stay balanced.

Uplifting Teas for Positivity

1. Lemon Balm Positivity Tea

- Steep 1 tablespoon dried lemon balm leaves in 1 cup boiling water for 10 minutes.
- Drink to calm anxiety and boost your mood.

2. Holy Basil (Tulsi) Adaptogenic Tea

- Brew 1 teaspoon dried tulsi leaves in 1 cup hot water for 10 minutes.
- Sip to improve mental clarity and reduce stress.

3. Peppermint and Rosemary Focus Tea

- Combine 1 teaspoon dried peppermint and 1/2 teaspoon dried rosemary in hot water.

- Drink to enhance focus and refresh your mind.

4. Rose and Hibiscus Mood-Lifting Tea

- Steep 1 teaspoon each of dried rose petals and hibiscus flowers in boiling water.
- Sip to uplift your mood and brighten your day.

5. Green Tea and Lemon Energy Tea

- Brew 1 teaspoon green tea with a slice of fresh lemon.
- Drink for a gentle boost of energy and mental clarity.

6. Chamomile and Lemon Zest Anti-Anxiety Tea

- Brew 1 teaspoon dried chamomile flowers with fresh lemon zest.
- Drink to reduce tension and promote a positive outlook.

7. Ginger and Orange Sunshine Tea

- Simmer 1 teaspoon grated ginger and a slice of orange peel in 2 cups water for 10 minutes.
- Drink to warm your spirit and energize your body.

8. Lavender and Lemon Balm Relaxation Tea

- Combine 1/2 teaspoon dried lavender with 1 teaspoon lemon balm in hot water.
- Sip to soothe anxiety and restore emotional balance.

9. Nettle and Peppermint Energizing Tea

- Steep 1 teaspoon dried nettle and 1 teaspoon dried peppermint in hot water for 10 minutes.

- Drink to boost energy and sharpen focus.

10. Matcha and Mint Brain-Boost Tea

- Whisk 1 teaspoon matcha powder into warm water with a few fresh mint leaves.
- Drink for sustained mental clarity and focus.

Herbal Tinctures for Mental Clarity and Emotional Balance

11. Ashwagandha Adaptogenic Tincture

- Take 1–2 droppers of ashwagandha tincture daily to support stress resilience and improve mood.

12. Lemon Balm Calming Tincture

- Take 1 dropper of lemon balm tincture during moments of anxiety or overwhelm to restore calm.

13. Rhodiola Energy and Focus Tincture

- Use 1 dropper of rhodiola tincture when you need a mental energy boost or help with focus.

14. Holy Basil Stress-Reducing Tincture

- Take 1 dropper of tulsi tincture daily to balance emotions and promote mental clarity.

15. Passionflower Relaxation Tincture

- Use 1 dropper of passionflower tincture when you feel tense or need help unwinding.

16. Skullcap Nervine Tincture

- Take 1–2 droppers of skullcap tincture to ease restlessness and emotional overload.

17. Ginseng Energy Tincture

- Use 1 dropper of ginseng tincture to combat fatigue and improve cognitive function.

18. St. John's Wort Mood-Boosting Tincture

- Take 1 dropper of St. John's Wort tincture daily to help ease mild depression and uplift your mood.

19. Milky Oat Nervous System Tincture

- Take 1 dropper of milky oat tincture to soothe frazzled nerves and restore focus.

20. Rose Petal Emotional Balance Tincture

- Use 1 dropper of rose petal tincture during moments of sadness or emotional stress to feel centered.

Aromatherapy Blends for Positivity and Focus

21. Lavender and Orange Uplifting Diffuser Blend

- Add 4 drops lavender oil and 3 drops sweet orange oil to your diffuser.

- Use to create a cheerful, calming atmosphere.

22. Peppermint and Rosemary Mental Clarity Blend

- Combine 3 drops peppermint oil with 2 drops rosemary oil.

- Diffuse to improve focus and clear mental fog.

23. Lemon and Geranium Happy Blend

- Mix 3 drops lemon oil with 3 drops geranium oil.
- Diffuse for a mood-lifting, energizing effect.

24. Frankincense and Sandalwood Centering Blend

- Add 4 drops frankincense oil and 2 drops sandalwood oil to your diffuser.
- Use during meditation or quiet moments for emotional grounding.

25. Ylang-Ylang and Grapefruit Energy Blend

- Combine 3 drops ylang-ylang oil with 3 drops grapefruit oil.
- Diffuse to balance emotions and uplift your energy.

26. Lavender and Peppermint Stress Relief Blend

- Mix 4 drops lavender oil with 2 drops peppermint oil.
- Diffuse to release tension and restore mental clarity.

27. Jasmine and Vanilla Comforting Blend

- Add 3 drops jasmine oil and 3 drops vanilla oil to your diffuser.
- Use to create a warm, soothing environment.

28. Clary Sage and Orange Creativity Blend

- Combine 3 drops clary sage oil with 3 drops sweet orange oil.
- Diffuse to inspire creativity and improve focus.

29. Eucalyptus and Lemon Refreshing Blend

- Mix 3 drops eucalyptus oil with 3 drops lemon oil.
- Diffuse to energize your space and clear mental clutter.

30. Patchouli and Lavender Relaxation Blend

- Add 3 drops patchouli oil and 3 drops lavender oil to your diffuser.
- Use to calm your mind and lift your mood after a stressful day.

PART 5: FAMILY AND WOMEN'S WELLNESS

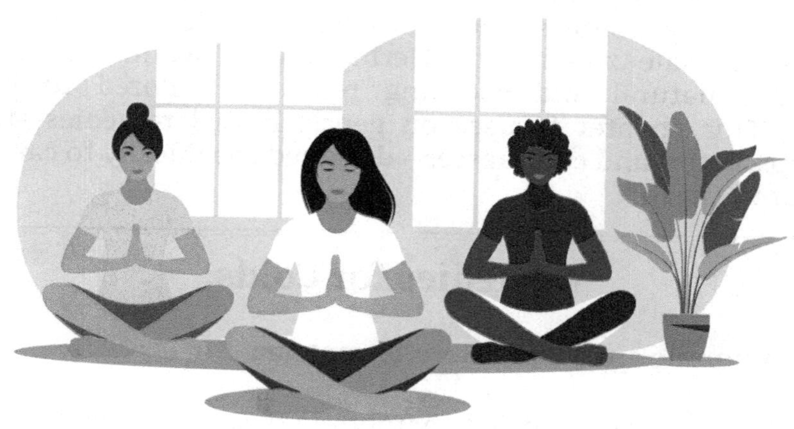

5.1 GENTLE REMEDIES FOR CHILDREN

Children often face common ailments like colds, fevers, and tummy troubles, but their smaller bodies require gentle and safe treatments. Herbs can be wonderful allies, offering natural and soothing remedies tailored to little ones. This chapter focuses on gentle herbal remedies—teas, syrups, baths, and compresses—designed specifically to care for children's health.

Remedies for Colds

1. Chamomile and Honey Sore Throat Tea

- Steep 1 teaspoon dried chamomile flowers in 1 cup boiling water for 5–7 minutes.
- Add 1 teaspoon honey (for children over 1 year old).
- Serve warm to soothe sore throats and calm restlessness.

2. Elderberry Syrup for Colds

- Simmer 1/2 cup dried elderberries in 2 cups water for 20 minutes.
- Strain, cool, and mix with 1/4 cup honey.
- Give 1 teaspoon daily as a preventative or 2–3 times daily during a cold.

3. Lemon Balm Cold Comfort Tea

- Brew 1 teaspoon dried lemon balm leaves in 1 cup hot water for 5–7 minutes.
- Serve warm to reduce fever, ease anxiety, and soothe cold symptoms.

4. Onion Vapor for Stuffy Nose

- Slice a raw onion and place it near your child's bed.
- The vapors help clear nasal congestion naturally while they sleep.

5. Peppermint Steam for Sinus Relief

- Add 1 teaspoon dried peppermint leaves to a bowl of hot water.
- Let your child inhale the steam (supervise closely) to clear sinuses.

6. Ginger Foot Bath for Congestion

- Add 2 tablespoons grated ginger to a basin of warm water.
- Let your child soak their feet for 10–15 minutes to improve circulation and relieve congestion.

7. Eucalyptus Chest Rub

- Mix 1/4 cup coconut oil with 3 drops eucalyptus essential oil (diluted for children).
- Rub gently onto their chest to ease breathing.

8. Elderflower and Rosehip Immune Tea

- Brew 1 teaspoon dried elderflowers and 1 teaspoon dried

rosehips in hot water for 5 minutes.

- Serve warm to boost the immune system and reduce fever.

9. Warm Compress for Earaches

- Soak a cloth in warm chamomile tea, wring it out, and place it over the affected ear.
- Relieves pain and reduces inflammation.

10. Thyme Cough Syrup

- Simmer 1 teaspoon dried thyme in 1 cup water for 10 minutes.
- Strain and mix with 1 teaspoon honey. Give 1–2 teaspoons to calm coughs (for children over 1 year old).

Remedies for Fevers

11. Chamomile and Lavender Fever Bath

- Add 1 tablespoon dried chamomile and 1 tablespoon dried lavender to a bowl of hot water. Let steep for 10 minutes, then pour into a warm bath.
- Bathe your child to calm their body and help reduce fever.

12. Lemon Sock Treatment

- Soak cotton socks in fresh lemon juice, wring them out, and place them on your child's feet. Cover with dry socks.
- This draws heat away from the body and reduces fever naturally.

13. Peppermint Cooling Compress

- Brew 1 cup peppermint tea, let it cool, and soak a cloth in the tea.
- Apply to your child's forehead or back of the neck to cool them down.

14. Elderflower Fever Tea

- Brew 1 teaspoon dried elderflowers in 1 cup boiling water for 5–7 minutes.
- Serve to encourage sweating and help the body break a fever.

15. Apple Cider Vinegar Bath

- Add 1/4 cup apple cider vinegar to a lukewarm bath.
- Bathe your child to naturally lower a fever and balance their body temperature.

16. Ginger and Lemon Fever Tea

- Simmer 1 teaspoon grated ginger in 1 cup water for 5 minutes. Add a squeeze of lemon and honey (if age-appropriate).
- Drink warm to reduce chills and improve circulation.

17. Basil Fever Relief Tea

- Steep 1 teaspoon dried basil leaves in hot water for 5 minutes.
- Serve to help bring down fever and support immunity.

18. Calendula and Chamomile Fever Compress

- Brew 1 tablespoon each of calendula and chamomile in 2 cups hot water. Let cool, soak a cloth, and place on the child's forehead to soothe fever.

19. Cool Peppermint and Lavender Mist

- Combine 1/4 cup distilled water with 2 drops peppermint essential oil and 2 drops lavender essential oil in a spray bottle.

- Lightly mist the air around your child to cool and calm them.

20. Yarrow Fever Tea

- Steep 1 teaspoon dried yarrow in 1 cup boiling water for 5 minutes.

- Serve warm to encourage sweating and gently break a fever.

Remedies for Digestive Troubles

21. Chamomile and Fennel Digestive Tea

- Steep 1 teaspoon dried chamomile flowers and 1/2 teaspoon crushed fennel seeds in 1 cup hot water for 5–7 minutes.

- Serve to relieve gas, bloating, and tummy aches.

22. Ginger Tummy Soother

- Mix 1/4 teaspoon grated fresh ginger with 1 teaspoon honey (if age-appropriate) in warm water.

- Give to ease nausea or an upset stomach.

23. Peppermint Tummy Calming Tea

- Brew 1 teaspoon dried peppermint leaves in 1 cup hot water for 5 minutes.

- Serve to soothe an upset stomach and reduce cramping.

24. Dill Seed Colic Tea

- Simmer 1/2 teaspoon crushed dill seeds in 1 cup water for 5 minutes.
- Cool and give small sips to relieve colic or gas pains.

25. Banana and Honey Digestive Smoothie

- Blend 1 ripe banana with 1 teaspoon honey and a splash of almond milk.
- Serve to calm an upset stomach and restore energy.

26. Slippery Elm Bark Digestive Paste

- Mix 1/2 teaspoon slippery elm powder with a little water to form a paste.
- Feed to your child to coat the stomach and relieve digestive discomfort.

27. Apple Cider Vinegar Digestive Tonic

- Mix 1 teaspoon apple cider vinegar with 1 cup water and a touch of honey (if age-appropriate).
- Give small sips to ease bloating or indigestion.

28. Warm Rice Water for Diarrhea

- Boil 1/2 cup rice in 2 cups water for 10 minutes. Strain and cool the liquid.
- Offer small sips to calm the stomach and replace lost fluids.

29. Cinnamon and Ginger Digestive Aid

- Simmer 1/4 teaspoon cinnamon and 1/4 teaspoon grated ginger in 1 cup water.
- Cool and serve small amounts to ease nausea and support digestion.

30. Probiotic Yogurt Snack

- Serve plain yogurt with a drizzle of honey (if age-appropriate).
- Helps restore gut health after digestive troubles.

5.2 WOMEN'S HEALTH

Women's bodies experience unique cycles and transitions, from monthly hormonal fluctuations to the profound changes of menopause. Herbs have been used for centuries to support women's health, offering relief from menstrual discomfort, helping balance hormones, and easing the symptoms of menopause. This chapter provides remedies to care for your body at every stage.

Remedies for Menstrual Relief

1. Ginger and Cinnamon Cramp-Relief Tea

- Simmer 1 teaspoon grated ginger and 1/2 teaspoon cinnamon powder in 1 cup water for 10 minutes.
- Drink to reduce inflammation, ease cramps, and promote circulation.

2. Raspberry Leaf Uterine Tonic Tea

- Brew 1 tablespoon dried raspberry leaf in 1 cup boiling water for 10 minutes.
- Drink daily during your cycle to tone the uterus and ease menstrual flow.

3. Chamomile and Lavender Relaxation Tea

- Combine 1 teaspoon dried chamomile with 1/2 teaspoon dried lavender in hot water.

- Sip to calm muscle spasms, reduce stress, and ease PMS-related mood swings.

4. Peppermint and Fennel Bloating Tea

- Brew 1 teaspoon dried peppermint leaves with 1/2 teaspoon crushed fennel seeds in boiling water.
- Drink to relieve bloating and digestive discomfort during menstruation.

5. Cramp Bark Tincture for Painful Cramps

- Take 1 dropper of cramp bark tincture (available commercially or homemade) every few hours during intense cramps.
- Helps relax uterine muscles and reduce pain.

6. Warm Castor Oil Compress for Cramps

- Soak a cloth in warm castor oil, place it on your lower abdomen, and cover with a towel.
- Leave for 20–30 minutes to relieve menstrual cramps naturally.

7. Yarrow and Chamomile Menstrual Soothing Tea

- Brew 1 teaspoon dried yarrow and 1 teaspoon dried chamomile in hot water.
- Sip to ease heavy bleeding and calm the nervous system.

8. Turmeric Golden Milk for Cramps

- Mix 1/2 teaspoon turmeric powder into warm milk (dairy or plant-based) with a pinch of black pepper and honey.
- Drink to reduce inflammation and ease muscle pain.

9. Magnesium-Rich Nettle and Oat Straw Tea

- Steep 1 tablespoon dried nettle with 1 tablespoon dried oat straw in hot water for 15 minutes.
- Drink to relax muscles and replenish nutrients during your cycle.

10. Rose Petal and Lemon Balm Mood Tea

- Brew 1 teaspoon dried rose petals with 1 teaspoon dried lemon balm in hot water.
- Sip to soothe emotional tension and promote a sense of calm.

Remedies for Hormonal Balance

11. Vitex (Chasteberry) Hormonal Balancing Tincture

- Take 1 dropper of vitex tincture daily in the morning.
- Helps regulate cycles, balance hormones, and reduce PMS symptoms.

12. Ashwagandha Adaptogenic Tea

- Brew 1 teaspoon ashwagandha powder in hot water or milk.
- Drink daily to reduce cortisol levels and improve hormonal balance.

13. Maca Root Energy Smoothie

- Blend 1 teaspoon maca powder with almond milk, a banana, and a dash of cinnamon.
- Drink to support hormonal health and boost energy levels.

14. Red Clover and Alfalfa Hormonal Support Tea

- Steep 1 teaspoon dried red clover and 1 teaspoon dried alfalfa in hot water for 10 minutes.
- Drink to support estrogen balance and improve overall hormonal health.

15. Holy Basil (Tulsi) Stress Relief Tea

- Brew 1 teaspoon dried tulsi in boiling water for 10 minutes.
- Drink to reduce cortisol and promote hormonal balance.

16. Licorice Root Tea for Hormonal Support

- Simmer 1 teaspoon dried licorice root in 1 cup water for 10 minutes.
- Drink in moderation (avoid if you have high blood pressure) to support adrenal health and balance hormones.

17. Evening Primrose Oil for PMS

- Take 1,000–2,000 mg evening primrose oil capsules daily.
- Helps reduce PMS symptoms like breast tenderness and mood swings.

18. Cinnamon and Ginger Hormonal Support Tea

- Simmer 1/2 teaspoon cinnamon and 1 teaspoon fresh ginger in water for 10 minutes.
- Drink to regulate blood sugar, which helps balance hormones.

19. Fenugreek Seed Hormonal Support Tea

- Simmer 1 teaspoon fenugreek seeds in 1 cup water for 10

minutes.

- Sip to support healthy hormone levels and promote balance.

20. Reishi Mushroom Adaptogenic Tonic

- Simmer 1 teaspoon dried reishi mushroom in 2 cups water for 30 minutes.
- Drink daily to regulate stress hormones and boost overall health.

Remedies for Menopause

21. Sage and Lemon Balm Hot Flash Tea

- Brew 1 teaspoon dried sage with 1 teaspoon lemon balm in hot water.
- Sip to reduce the intensity of hot flashes and calm the mind.

22. Black Cohosh Tincture for Menopausal Symptoms

- Take 1–2 droppers of black cohosh tincture daily.
- Supports hormone balance and reduces hot flashes, night sweats, and mood swings.

23. Red Clover and Hibiscus Hormonal Tea

- Steep 1 teaspoon dried red clover with 1 teaspoon hibiscus flowers in boiling water.
- Drink to support estrogen balance and reduce menopausal symptoms.

24. Peppermint and Lavender Cooling Spray

- Mix 1/4 cup distilled water with 2 drops peppermint

essential oil and 2 drops lavender essential oil in a spray bottle.

- Mist onto your skin during hot flashes for cooling relief.

25. Dong Quai Hormonal Support Tea

- Simmer 1 teaspoon dried dong quai root in 2 cups water for 15 minutes.
- Drink to support hormonal balance and relieve menopausal symptoms.

26. Nettle and Horsetail Bone-Strengthening Tea

- Steep 1 tablespoon dried nettle with 1 tablespoon dried horsetail in boiling water.
- Drink to support bone density and reduce menopause-related bone loss.

27. Evening Primrose and Flaxseed Hormone Smoothie

- Blend 1 teaspoon ground flaxseed and 1 teaspoon evening primrose oil into a smoothie.
- Drink to support hormone health and reduce hot flashes.

28. Chamomile and Passionflower Menopause Tea

- Brew 1 teaspoon dried chamomile with 1 teaspoon dried passionflower in boiling water.
- Sip to reduce anxiety and promote restful sleep.

29. Ashwagandha Energy Restoring Tea

- Brew 1 teaspoon ashwagandha in milk or water.
- Drink daily to boost energy and reduce menopause-related

fatigue.

30. Lavender and Sage Relaxing Bath Soak

- Add 1/4 cup dried lavender and 1/4 cup dried sage to a warm bath.
- Soak for 20 minutes to ease muscle tension, calm the mind, and reduce menopause symptoms.

5.3 PREGNANCY AND POSTPARTUM CARE

Pregnancy and postpartum are transformative times for a woman's body, but they often come with challenges like nausea, fatigue, postpartum recovery, and lactation issues. Herbal remedies can provide gentle, natural support when chosen carefully, ensuring safety for both mother and baby. This chapter includes remedies tailored to support pregnancy and postpartum wellness.

Remedies for Pregnancy Nausea

1. Ginger Tea for Morning Sickness

- Simmer 1 teaspoon grated fresh ginger in 1 cup water for 5 minutes.
- Sip slowly to relieve nausea. (Drink no more than 2–3 cups per day during pregnancy.)

2. Lemon Balm Calming Tea

- Brew 1 teaspoon dried lemon balm leaves in hot water for 10 minutes.
- Drink to ease nausea and reduce anxiety.

3. Peppermint Inhalation for Nausea Relief

- Add 2 drops peppermint essential oil to a bowl of hot water.

- Inhale deeply to ease nausea (avoid internal use of peppermint oil during pregnancy).

4. Mint and Lemon Morning Sickness Tea

- Steep 1 teaspoon dried peppermint leaves with 1 teaspoon fresh lemon juice in hot water.
- Drink to reduce queasiness.

5. Apple and Ginger Digestive Snack

- Dip thin apple slices in fresh ginger juice and snack on them to settle your stomach.

6. Fennel Seed Tea for Digestive Relief

- Brew 1/2 teaspoon crushed fennel seeds in hot water for 10 minutes.
- Sip to reduce nausea and bloating.

7. Chamomile and Honey Nausea Soother

- Steep 1 teaspoon dried chamomile in hot water for 5 minutes.
- Add honey and drink to relax and reduce nausea.

8. Cardamom and Clove Digestive Tea

- Simmer 2 cardamom pods and 2 cloves in 1 cup water for 5 minutes.
- Strain and sip to relieve an upset stomach.

9. Raspberry Leaf Gentle Tonic

- Brew 1 teaspoon dried raspberry leaf in hot water for 10 minutes.

- Sip slowly to support digestion and gently tone the uterus.

10. Lemon and Ginger Popsicles

- Combine fresh lemon juice with grated ginger and honey, then freeze in popsicle molds.
- Suck on them during bouts of nausea for soothing relief.

Postpartum Recovery Remedies

11. Arnica Homeopathic Remedy for Pain Relief

- Take arnica tablets (homeopathic remedy) to reduce swelling and ease postpartum soreness.

12. Calendula Sitz Bath for Healing

- Brew 2 tablespoons dried calendula flowers in hot water for 10 minutes, then add to a shallow sitz bath.
- Use to promote healing of perineal tears or stitches.

13. Raspberry Leaf Uterine Recovery Tea

- Brew 1 tablespoon dried raspberry leaf in hot water for 10 minutes.
- Drink 2–3 cups daily to support uterine recovery and reduce postpartum bleeding.

14. Witch Hazel Pads for Soreness

- Soak cotton pads in pure witch hazel and refrigerate.
- Place on the perineal area to reduce swelling and soothe soreness.

15. Turmeric and Honey Anti-Inflammatory Tonic

- Mix 1/2 teaspoon turmeric powder with honey and warm milk (dairy or plant-based).
- Drink to reduce inflammation and support overall recovery.

16. Chamomile and Lavender Sleep Tea

- Brew 1 teaspoon dried chamomile with 1/2 teaspoon lavender in hot water.
- Sip to promote relaxation and restful sleep during postpartum recovery.

17. St. John's Wort Mood Tea

- Brew 1 teaspoon dried St. John's Wort in hot water for 10 minutes.
- Drink to support emotional balance and ease postpartum blues.

18. Nettle and Oat Straw Nourishing Tea

- Combine 1 tablespoon nettle with 1 tablespoon oat straw and steep in hot water for 10–15 minutes.
- Drink to replenish minerals and energy levels after childbirth.

19. Fenugreek and Ginger Recovery Soup

- Add 1 teaspoon fenugreek seeds and 1 teaspoon grated ginger to a vegetable or chicken broth.
- Sip to support recovery and digestion.

20. Bone Broth for Strength and Healing

- Simmer bones with garlic, ginger, and vegetables for several hours.

- Drink daily to nourish the body, support healing, and improve energy.

Remedies for Lactation Support

21. Fenugreek and Fennel Milk Supply Tea

- Simmer 1 teaspoon fenugreek seeds and 1/2 teaspoon fennel seeds in 2 cups water for 10 minutes.

- Strain and drink twice daily to enhance milk supply.

22. Oatmeal and Flaxseed Lactation Booster

- Cook oatmeal and stir in 1 tablespoon ground flaxseed and honey.

- Eat daily to support milk production.

23. Blessed Thistle and Alfalfa Lactation Tea

- Brew 1 teaspoon dried blessed thistle with 1 teaspoon alfalfa in hot water for 10 minutes.

- Drink to encourage milk flow.

24. Goat's Rue Milk-Producing Tincture

- Take 1 dropper of goat's rue tincture (available commercially) twice daily.

- Helps stimulate milk production.

25. Fennel and Lemon Water Hydration Tonic

- Add fresh lemon slices and 1 teaspoon fennel seeds to a pitcher of water.

- Sip throughout the day to stay hydrated and boost milk production.

26. Milk Thistle Lactation Support Tea

- Brew 1 teaspoon dried milk thistle seeds in hot water for 10 minutes.
- Drink daily to support milk supply.

27. Lactation Energy Balls

- Mix oats, flaxseed, almond butter, honey, and shredded coconut into a dough.
- Roll into balls and refrigerate. Eat as a nourishing lactation snack.

28. Brewer's Yeast Smoothie for Milk Supply

- Blend 1 teaspoon brewer's yeast with almond milk, a banana, and a handful of spinach.
- Drink to boost energy and milk production.

29. Nettle and Oat Milk Tea for Nourishment

- Steep 1 tablespoon dried nettle with 1 cup oat milk for 10 minutes.
- Drink to replenish iron and improve lactation.

30. Warm Compress for Milk Flow

- Soak a cloth in warm water, wring it out, and place it on the breasts before nursing.
- Helps stimulate milk flow and ease engorgement.

PART 6: SEASONAL AND LIFESTYLE HERBALISM

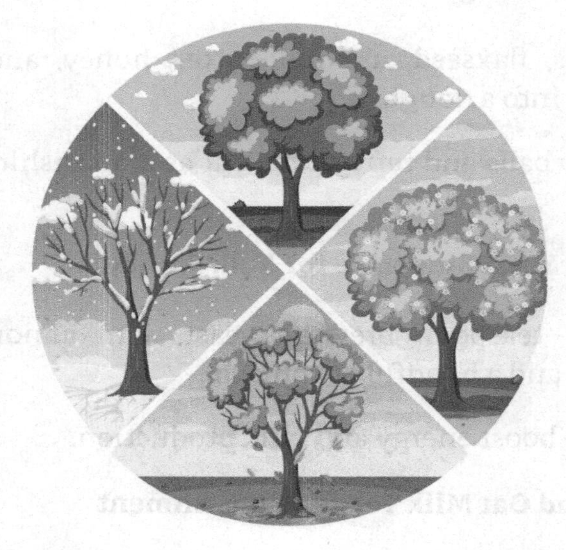

6.1 SEASONAL REMEDIES

Each season brings its own challenges and opportunities for wellness. In spring, we focus on renewal and detoxification. Summer calls for cooling herbs to beat the heat. Autumn emphasizes boosting immunity to prepare for colder months, while winter brings the need for warming, comforting remedies. This chapter provides herbal remedies to help you stay in harmony with the seasons and support your body's changing needs.

Spring Cleansing Remedies

1. Dandelion Detox Tea

- Brew 1 tablespoon dried dandelion root in 2 cups water for 10 minutes.
- Drink daily to flush out toxins and support liver health.

2. Nettle Infusion for Energy

- Steep 2 tablespoons dried nettle in 1 quart hot water for 4–8 hours.
- Drink to replenish minerals and energy after winter.

3. Burdock and Mint Cleansing Tea

- Brew 1 teaspoon dried burdock root and 1 teaspoon peppermint in 1 cup boiling water.
- Sip to support kidney health and freshen your system.

4. Lemon Ginger Morning Tonic

- Mix the juice of 1 lemon with 1 teaspoon grated ginger in warm water.
- Drink first thing in the morning to aid digestion and detoxification.

5. Parsley and Cilantro Detox Smoothie

- Blend 1 handful parsley, 1 handful cilantro, 1/2 cucumber, and lemon juice with water.
- Drink to support kidney and liver detox.

6. Red Clover Tea for Blood Purification

- Steep 1 teaspoon dried red clover blossoms in 1 cup boiling water.
- Drink to cleanse the blood and improve circulation.

7. Calendula Lymphatic Cleansing Tea

- Brew 1 teaspoon dried calendula flowers in 1 cup hot water.
- Sip to support the lymphatic system's detox process.

8. Beet and Apple Liver Tonic

- Blend 1 beet, 1 apple, and 1/2 lemon into a smoothie.
- Drink to rejuvenate your liver and digestion.

9. Milk Thistle Tea for Liver Support

- Brew 1 teaspoon milk thistle seeds in 1 cup hot water.
- Drink to protect and detoxify the liver.

10. Spring Cleansing Vegetable Soup

- Simmer dandelion greens, parsley, garlic, and celery in a vegetable broth.
- Enjoy to gently detox your body and nourish with minerals.

Summer Cooling Remedies

11. Hibiscus and Peppermint Iced Tea

- Brew 1 tablespoon dried hibiscus flowers with 1 teaspoon dried peppermint in 4 cups hot water.
- Cool, add ice, and sweeten with honey for a refreshing drink.

12. Watermelon and Mint Cooler

- Blend watermelon chunks with fresh mint leaves and ice.
- Enjoy to stay hydrated and cool.

13. Aloe Vera Lemonade

- Mix 2 tablespoons fresh aloe vera gel with 1 cup lemonade.
- Drink to cool your body and soothe inflammation.

14. Rose and Cucumber Facial Mist

- Blend cucumber juice with rosewater and store in a spray bottle.
- Mist your face to cool and refresh your skin.

15. Chrysanthemum Tea for Summer Heat

- Brew 1 teaspoon dried chrysanthemum flowers in 1 cup hot water.

- Cool and sip to reduce internal heat and calm inflammation.

16. Lavender and Lemon Balm Cooling Tea

- Brew 1 teaspoon each of dried lavender and lemon balm in hot water.
- Chill and drink to cool the body and relax your mind.

17. Mint and Lemon Infused Water

- Add fresh mint leaves and lemon slices to a pitcher of cold water.
- Sip throughout the day to stay hydrated.

18. Rose and Hibiscus Popsicles

- Brew a strong tea with rose petals and hibiscus flowers, add honey, and freeze in popsicle molds.

19. Coconut Water and Lime Rehydration Drink

- Mix coconut water with fresh lime juice.
- Drink to replenish electrolytes and cool your body.

20. Cucumber Aloe Face Mask

- Blend fresh cucumber with aloe vera gel.
- Apply to your face for 15 minutes to reduce redness and cool your skin.

Autumn Immunity Remedies

21. Elderberry Immune Syrup

- Simmer 1/2 cup dried elderberries with 2 cups water for 30 minutes.

- Strain, cool, and mix with honey. Take 1 teaspoon daily.

22. Garlic and Honey Immune Booster

- Mince fresh garlic and mix with raw honey.
- Take 1 teaspoon daily to ward off colds.

23. Fire Cider

- Infuse apple cider vinegar with garlic, ginger, horseradish, and cayenne for 4 weeks.
- Take 1 tablespoon daily for immune support.

24. Echinacea Tea for Immunity

- Steep 1 teaspoon dried echinacea in 1 cup boiling water.
- Sip to boost your immune system.

25. Turmeric and Ginger Immune Tonic

- Simmer 1/2 teaspoon turmeric powder and 1 teaspoon grated ginger in water.
- Add honey and lemon to drink.

26. Rosehip and Hibiscus Vitamin C Tea

- Steep 1 teaspoon each of dried rosehips and hibiscus in hot water.
- Drink for a boost of antioxidants and vitamin C.

27. Thyme Steam Inhalation

- Add 1 teaspoon dried thyme to a bowl of hot water.

- Inhale the steam to clear sinuses and prevent infections.

28. Elderflower Fever Tea

- Brew 1 teaspoon dried elderflowers in hot water.
- Sip to reduce fevers and boost immunity.

29. Ginger and Lemon Foot Bath

- Add grated ginger and lemon slices to a basin of warm water.
- Soak your feet to detox and improve circulation.

30. Immune-Boosting Soup

- Simmer garlic, ginger, carrots, and turmeric in a broth.
- Add parsley and sip to strengthen immunity.

Winter Warmth Remedies

31. Spiced Golden Milk

- Heat 1 cup milk (dairy or plant-based) with 1/2 teaspoon turmeric, a pinch of cinnamon, and black pepper.
- Sweeten with honey and sip to warm your body.

32. Ginger and Cinnamon Warming Tea

- Simmer 1 teaspoon grated ginger and 1 cinnamon stick in 2 cups water.
- Sip to improve circulation and fight chills.

33. Elderberry and Clove Cough Syrup

- Simmer elderberries with cloves, ginger, and honey to make a syrup.

- Take 1 teaspoon for cough relief.

34. Rosemary and Thyme Respiratory Steam

- Add 1 teaspoon each of rosemary and thyme to a bowl of hot water.
- Inhale deeply to clear congestion.

35. Peppermint and Eucalyptus Chest Rub

- Mix 1/4 cup coconut oil with 5 drops eucalyptus oil and 3 drops peppermint oil.
- Massage onto your chest for relief from colds.

36. Clove and Orange Aromatic Tea

- Simmer orange peels with cloves and a cinnamon stick.
- Sip for a warming, immune-boosting drink.

37. Sage and Honey Sore Throat Tea

- Brew 1 teaspoon dried sage in hot water and add honey.
- Drink to soothe a sore throat.

38. Bone Broth with Herbs

- Simmer bones with garlic, rosemary, thyme, and ginger for hours.
- Drink to warm your body and strengthen immunity.

39. Spiced Apple Cider

- Heat apple cider with cinnamon sticks, cloves, and orange

slices.

- Sip for a cozy, warming drink.

40. Ginger and Mustard Seed Foot Soak

- Add 1 tablespoon grated ginger and 1 teaspoon mustard seeds to warm water.
- Soak your feet to improve circulation and warm your body.

6.2 HERBS FOR ACTIVE LIFESTYLES

Active lifestyles, whether from physical activity or the demands of a busy schedule, require recovery support, energy replenishment, and stress management. Herbs can naturally assist with boosting stamina, reducing inflammation, relieving muscle soreness, and improving endurance. This chapter includes remedies to help you stay energized, recover faster, and maintain balance.

Energy-Boosting Remedies

1. Ashwagandha Energy Latte

- Mix 1 teaspoon ashwagandha powder with warm milk (dairy or plant-based), honey, and a pinch of cinnamon.
- Drink daily to boost energy levels and reduce fatigue caused by physical or mental stress.

2. Matcha Mint Energizing Tea

- Brew 1 teaspoon matcha powder with fresh mint leaves in warm water.
- Sip to improve stamina and mental clarity during busy days.

3. Ginseng and Lemon Energy Shot

- Brew 1 teaspoon powdered ginseng in warm water with

fresh lemon juice.

- Drink to naturally enhance endurance and energy.

4. Nettle and Peppermint Mineral-Rich Tea

- Steep 1 tablespoon dried nettle leaves and 1 teaspoon dried peppermint in hot water.
- Drink to replenish minerals and maintain energy levels.

5. Adaptogenic Smoothie

- Blend 1 teaspoon maca powder with almond milk, a banana, and a dash of cinnamon.
- Perfect as a pre-workout or morning energy drink.

6. Holy Basil (Tulsi) Stress Tea

- Brew 1 teaspoon dried tulsi in hot water for 10 minutes.
- Drink daily to reduce cortisol levels and keep energy balanced.

7. Eleuthero (Siberian Ginseng) Stamina Tea

- Brew 1 teaspoon eleuthero root in hot water for 15 minutes.
- Sip to improve physical endurance and reduce fatigue.

8. Rosemary and Lemon Energizing Tonic

- Steep 1 teaspoon fresh rosemary in hot water with a slice of lemon.
- Drink to stimulate circulation and refresh your mind.

9. Chia Seed Electrolyte Drink

- Soak 1 tablespoon chia seeds in 2 cups water, add a squeeze of lime juice and a pinch of sea salt.
- Drink to rehydrate and energize after exercise.

10. Ginger and Turmeric Energy Tea

- Simmer 1 teaspoon grated ginger and 1/2 teaspoon turmeric in 2 cups water for 10 minutes.
- Drink to reduce inflammation and improve stamina.

Recovery Remedies for Athletes

11. Arnica and St. John's Wort Massage Oil

- Infuse arnica and St. John's Wort flowers in olive oil for 4 weeks, strain, and use as a massage oil.
- Apply to sore muscles to reduce inflammation and speed recovery.

12. Epsom Salt and Lavender Recovery Bath

- Add 1 cup Epsom salts and 10 drops lavender essential oil to a warm bath.
- Soak for 20 minutes to relax sore muscles and restore magnesium levels.

13. Nettle and Oat Straw Mineral Recovery Tea

- Steep 1 tablespoon dried nettle with 1 tablespoon oat straw in hot water for 10 minutes.
- Drink post-workout to replenish lost minerals.

14. Tart Cherry Juice for Muscle Recovery

- Drink 1/2 cup tart cherry juice daily to reduce muscle soreness and inflammation.

15. Comfrey Poultice for Sore Muscles

- Crush fresh comfrey leaves into a paste and apply to sore muscles or bruises.
- Cover with a cloth and leave on for 20 minutes to reduce pain and swelling.

16. Licorice Root and Ginger Recovery Tea

- Brew 1 teaspoon dried licorice root with 1 teaspoon grated ginger in hot water.
- Sip to reduce inflammation and soothe post-workout fatigue.

17. Devil's Claw Pain Relief Tea

- Simmer 1 teaspoon dried devil's claw root in 2 cups water for 10 minutes.
- Drink to relieve joint and muscle pain after strenuous activity.

18. Calendula and Chamomile Soothing Bath

- Brew 1 tablespoon dried calendula and 1 tablespoon dried chamomile in hot water, strain, and add to your bath.
- Soak to reduce inflammation and relax tired muscles.

19. Magnesium-Rich Bone Broth

- Simmer bones with garlic, ginger, and turmeric for several hours.

- Sip to replenish nutrients and support muscle recovery.

20. Fenugreek Muscle Soothing Paste

- Make a paste with fenugreek seed powder and warm water, and apply to sore areas.
- Leave for 15 minutes to reduce inflammation and muscle tension.

Stress and Balance Remedies for Busy Lives

21. Lemon Balm Relaxation Tea

- Brew 1 tablespoon dried lemon balm leaves in 1 cup hot water.
- Sip to ease tension and improve focus during stressful days.

22. Passionflower Calm Tincture

- Take 1 dropper of passionflower tincture in water when feeling overwhelmed.
- Helps calm the mind and relieve anxiety.

23. Lavender and Peppermint Stress Relief Mist

- Combine 1/4 cup distilled water with 5 drops lavender oil and 3 drops peppermint oil in a spray bottle.
- Mist onto your face or around your space for instant relaxation.

24. Chamomile and Rose Calming Tea

- Brew 1 teaspoon dried chamomile with 1 teaspoon dried rose petals in hot water.

- Sip to promote emotional balance and calm nerves.

25. Adaptogenic Rhodiola Energy Tincture

- Take 1 dropper of rhodiola tincture daily to improve mental clarity and physical endurance during busy days.

26. Ashwagandha and Holy Basil Tea for Adrenal Support

- Combine 1 teaspoon each of ashwagandha and tulsi in hot water.

- Sip to support adrenal glands and restore balance.

27. Skullcap Nervine Relaxation Tea

- Steep 1 teaspoon dried skullcap leaves in hot water for 10 minutes.

- Drink to soothe frazzled nerves after a hectic day.

28. Lemon and Ginger Stress Relief Water

- Add slices of fresh lemon and ginger to a pitcher of water.

- Sip to stay hydrated while calming your digestive system.

29. Probiotic Herbal Yogurt Bowl

- Mix plain yogurt with fresh mint, honey, and a sprinkle of chia seeds.

- Eat to support gut health and maintain energy during busy periods.

30. Holy Basil and Lavender Sleep Tea

- Brew 1 teaspoon tulsi with 1/2 teaspoon dried lavender flowers in hot water.

- Drink before bed to calm your mind and promote restful sleep.

6.3 DETOX AND RENEWAL

Cleansing isn't just about eliminating toxins—it's also about refreshing your body, mind, and spirit. Herbal remedies can gently support your liver, kidneys, digestion, and lymphatic system while helping you feel revitalized and clear-headed. This chapter offers herbal teas, tonics, and simple detox remedies to help you renew your energy and achieve a sense of balance.

Herbal Teas for Detox and Cleansing

1. Dandelion Root Liver Detox Tea

- Simmer 1 teaspoon dried dandelion root in 2 cups water for 10 minutes.
- Sip daily to support liver function and promote toxin removal.

2. Nettle and Peppermint Mineral Detox Tea

- Brew 1 tablespoon dried nettle with 1 teaspoon dried peppermint in hot water for 10 minutes.
- Drink to replenish minerals and flush toxins.

3. Burdock Root Blood Cleanser Tea

- Simmer 1 teaspoon dried burdock root in 2 cups water for 15 minutes.
- Sip to purify the blood and support kidney health.

4. Red Clover Antioxidant Tea

- Steep 1 teaspoon dried red clover blossoms in hot water for 10 minutes.
- Drink to cleanse the blood and reduce inflammation.

5. Lemon and Ginger Morning Detox Tea

- Steep 1 teaspoon grated ginger in hot water with the juice of 1/2 lemon.
- Drink first thing in the morning to aid digestion and kick-start your metabolism.

6. Hibiscus and Rosehip Vitamin C Tea

- Brew 1 teaspoon each of dried hibiscus and rosehips in boiling water for 10 minutes.
- Drink to fight free radicals and hydrate while detoxing.

7. Milk Thistle Liver Support Tea

- Steep 1 teaspoon milk thistle seeds in hot water for 15 minutes.
- Sip to protect and regenerate liver cells.

8. Calendula and Lemon Balm Digestive Tea

- Brew 1 teaspoon dried calendula flowers with 1 teaspoon dried lemon balm.
- Drink to soothe digestion and promote lymphatic detoxification.

9. Yarrow and Peppermint Cleansing Tea

- Steep 1 teaspoon each of dried yarrow and peppermint

leaves in hot water.

- Sip to encourage gentle sweating and help the body eliminate toxins.

10. Green Tea with Mint Antioxidant Brew

- Brew 1 teaspoon green tea with a handful of fresh mint leaves.
- Sip for a cleansing boost of antioxidants and energy.

Herbal Tonics for Detox and Renewal

11. Apple Cider Vinegar Detox Tonic

- Mix 1 tablespoon apple cider vinegar with 1 cup warm water and 1 teaspoon honey.
- Drink daily to balance pH levels and support digestion.

12. Aloe Vera and Lemon Juice Cleanser

- Blend 2 tablespoons fresh aloe vera gel with the juice of 1/2 lemon and water.
- Drink to soothe digestion and cleanse your colon.

13. Cilantro and Lime Heavy Metal Detox Water

- Blend 1 handful cilantro with the juice of 1 lime and water.
- Drink to support the removal of heavy metals from the body.

14. Beet and Ginger Liver Tonic

- Blend 1 small beet, 1 teaspoon grated ginger, and 1 cup water into a smoothie.

- Sip to stimulate liver detox and improve digestion.

15. **Cucumber and Mint Hydration Tonic**

- Add sliced cucumber and fresh mint leaves to a pitcher of water.

- Sip throughout the day to stay hydrated and cool while detoxifying.

16. **Spirulina Detox Smoothie**

- Blend 1 teaspoon spirulina powder with almond milk, banana, and a handful of spinach.

- Drink to nourish and detoxify your cells.

17. **Ginger and Turmeric Inflammation Tonic**

- Simmer 1 teaspoon grated ginger and 1/2 teaspoon turmeric in water for 10 minutes.

- Add honey and lemon to sip for anti-inflammatory benefits.

18. **Dandelion and Parsley Kidney Tonic**

- Simmer 1 teaspoon dried dandelion root with fresh parsley in 2 cups water for 10 minutes.

- Drink to support kidney detoxification.

19. **Lemon Balm Stress-Relief Tonic**

- Brew 1 tablespoon dried lemon balm leaves in hot water and cool.

- Sip to calm the mind and detox from stress.

20. **Holy Basil (Tulsi) Renewal Tonic**

- Brew 1 teaspoon dried tulsi leaves in 1 cup hot water.
- Drink to reduce cortisol and rejuvenate body and mind.

Baths and Compresses for Detoxification

21. Epsom Salt and Lavender Detox Bath

- Add 1 cup Epsom salts and 10 drops lavender essential oil to a warm bath.
- Soak for 20 minutes to relax muscles and draw out toxins.

22. Apple Cider Vinegar Detox Bath

- Add 1/2 cup apple cider vinegar to a warm bath.
- Soak to balance your body's pH and soothe tired muscles.

23. Calendula and Chamomile Skin Detox Bath

- Brew 2 tablespoons each of dried calendula and chamomile in hot water, then add to your bath.
- Soak to calm skin and cleanse lymphatic pathways.

24. Ginger and Mustard Seed Foot Soak

- Add 1 tablespoon grated ginger and 1 teaspoon mustard seeds to warm water.
- Soak your feet to improve circulation and encourage sweating.

25. Rosemary and Sage Detox Steam

- Add 1 tablespoon each of rosemary and sage to a bowl of hot water.

- Inhale deeply to clear your sinuses and detoxify your respiratory system.

26. Nettle and Lemon Body Compress

- Brew 1 tablespoon dried nettle leaves in hot water, soak a cloth, and apply it to your chest or back.
- Use to nourish your skin and support detox.

27. Peppermint and Eucalyptus Detox Shower Mist

- Add 10 drops peppermint essential oil and 5 drops eucalyptus oil to your shower floor before stepping in.
- Let the steam cleanse your respiratory system.

28. Green Tea and Sea Salt Detox Bath

- Brew 2 cups strong green tea and add to a warm bath with 1/2 cup sea salt.
- Soak to draw out toxins and rejuvenate your skin.

29. Lemon and Baking Soda Detox Bath

- Add the juice of 1 lemon and 1/2 cup baking soda to a warm bath.
- Soak to alkalize your body and detoxify.

30. Chamomile and Rose Petal Facial Steam

- Add dried chamomile flowers and rose petals to a bowl of hot water.
- Steam your face to open pores and cleanse impurities.

PART 7: SPIRITUAL AND EMOTIONAL GROWTH

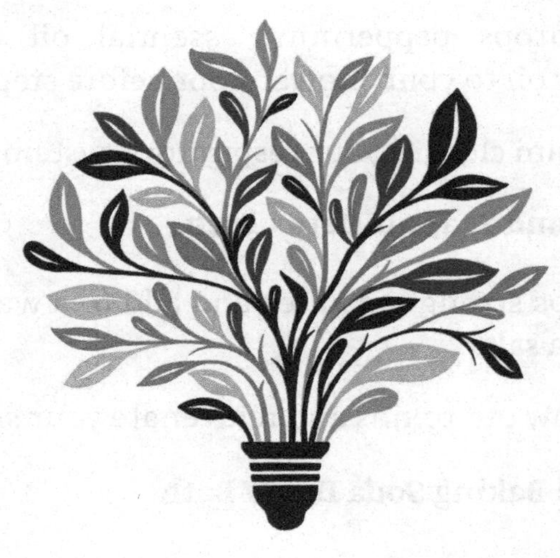

7.1 HARMONIOUS HOME

Creating a harmonious home means cultivating an environment that nurtures peace, balance, and positivity. These herbal remedies offer ways to cleanse negative energy, refresh your space with natural scents, and foster an atmosphere of love, abundance, and grounding. From smudging to simmer pots to herbal cleaning solutions, these remedies will help transform your home into a sanctuary.

Cleansing Your Space

1. White Sage Smudge Stick

- Light a bundle of dried white sage and waft the smoke through each room of your home.
- Focus on doorways, windows, and corners to clear out negative energy.

2. Rosemary and Lavender Protection Smudge

- Burn a bundle of dried rosemary and lavender to cleanse and protect your space.
- The combination clears negative energy while promoting a calming atmosphere.

3. Palo Santo Energy Clearing

- Light a stick of Palo Santo wood and let its fragrant smoke fill your home.

- Use to uplift energy and bring a sense of positivity to your space.

4. Bay Leaf Burning for Manifestation

- Write intentions (e.g., "peace," "abundance") on dried bay leaves.
- Burn the leaves in a safe dish to release stagnant energy and focus on your goals.

5. Salt and Sage Energy Clearing Spray

- Mix 1/4 cup distilled water, 1 tablespoon sea salt, and 5 drops sage essential oil in a spray bottle.
- Mist the air in each room to cleanse energy without smoke.

6. Thyme and Rosemary Floor Wash

- Brew a strong tea with thyme and rosemary, then mix it into warm mop water.
- Use to cleanse floors, particularly in high-traffic areas, for energetic clearing.

7. Eucalyptus Door Wreath

- Hang fresh eucalyptus over doorways to ward off negative energy and welcome harmony.

8. Lemon and Sage Disinfecting Wipe

- Infuse fresh lemon slices and sage leaves in vinegar for 2 weeks.
- Strain and use to wipe down counters and surfaces to clear both germs and bad vibes.

9. Peppermint and Lavender Air Refresh Mist

- Mix 1/4 cup distilled water with 5 drops peppermint essential oil and 5 drops lavender essential oil.
- Spray into the air to clear stagnant energy and refresh your home.

10. Mugwort Smoke for Dreamwork

- Burn dried mugwort in your bedroom before sleep.
- It's believed to cleanse the space and promote vivid, meaningful dreams.

Enhancing Your Atmosphere

11. Cinnamon and Orange Simmer Pot

- Simmer cinnamon sticks, orange peels, and cloves in water on the stove.
- Let the fragrant steam fill your home with warmth and positivity.

12. Lavender and Rosemary Simmer Pot

- Simmer dried lavender flowers and fresh rosemary sprigs in water.
- Use to create a calming and grounding atmosphere.

13. Rose Petal and Vanilla Potpourri

- Combine dried rose petals, vanilla beans, and lavender in a bowl.
- Place in living spaces to subtly scent the air and create an inviting ambiance.

14. Cedar and Juniper Incense

- Burn cedar and juniper incense to create a woodsy, grounding scent.
- Use during meditation or to feel connected to nature.

15. Mint and Eucalyptus Shower Steamer

- Hang a bundle of fresh mint and eucalyptus in your shower.
- The steam releases their refreshing scent, invigorating your mornings.

16. Lavender Drawer Sachets

- Fill small fabric pouches with dried lavender.
- Place in drawers or closets to subtly scent clothes and linens.

17. Sage and Citrus Stove Simmer

- Simmer fresh sage leaves and sliced lemons in water.
- Let the scent fill your home to uplift and refresh the atmosphere.

18. Jasmine and Vanilla Diffuser Blend

- Add 3 drops jasmine oil and 2 drops vanilla oil to a diffuser.
- Use to create a soothing and romantic atmosphere.

19. Peppermint and Rosemary Workspace Diffuser Blend

- Combine 3 drops peppermint oil with 3 drops rosemary oil.
- Diffuse in your workspace to boost focus and clarity.

20. Clove and Orange Festive Aroma Mist

- Mix 1/4 cup distilled water with 5 drops orange essential oil and 3 drops clove oil.
- Spray during holidays or gatherings for a festive scent.

Fostering Positivity and Protection

21. Basil and Mint Abundance Spray

- Infuse fresh basil and mint leaves in water for 24 hours.
- Strain and spray around your home to invite prosperity and positivity.

22. Rose Quartz and Lavender Bedroom Charm

- Place a bowl of dried lavender flowers and a rose quartz crystal on your nightstand.
- This combination promotes love, peace, and restful sleep.

23. Bay Leaves Under the Mat

- Place a few dried bay leaves under your welcome mat.
- Traditionally used to invite protection and good fortune into the home.

24. Cinnamon Stick Door Charm

- Tie cinnamon sticks together with red string and hang above your doorway.
- This is believed to protect your home from negative energy and welcome abundance.

25. Thyme and Rosemary Window Wash

- Brew a strong tea with thyme and rosemary, mix with vinegar, and use to clean windows.
- Helps cleanse the energy entering your home through natural light.

26. Lavender and Rose Love Candle

- Sprinkle dried lavender and rose petals around the base of a candle.
- Light it with the intention of inviting love and harmony into your home.

27. Chamomile and Basil Energy Jar

- Fill a small jar with dried chamomile and basil leaves.
- Place it in a central room to promote calmness and abundance.

28. Palo Santo Gratitude Ritual

- Light Palo Santo wood and walk through your home while expressing gratitude for each room.
- Use this practice to anchor positive energy.

29. Salt Water Cleansing Bowl

- Place a bowl of water with sea salt in the center of your home.
- Leave it overnight to absorb negative energy, then discard it the next day.

30. Eucalyptus and Rosemary Bedside Sachets

- Fill small bags with dried eucalyptus and rosemary, and

place them under your pillow or on your nightstand.

- Use to promote clarity and protection while you sleep.

7.2 EMOTIONAL BALANCE AND INNER PEACE

In a world full of distractions and demands, finding emotional balance and inner peace can feel like a challenge. Herbs offer gentle yet powerful support for calming anxiety, lifting the spirit, and grounding the mind. By incorporating herbal remedies into your daily rituals, you can create moments of tranquility, build resilience to life's stressors, and foster deeper self-awareness.

This chapter provides remedies to nurture your emotional health, help you navigate difficult times, and cultivate lasting inner peace. From soothing teas to aromatherapy blends and mindfulness practices, these remedies offer practical ways to restore balance and reconnect with your inner self.

Herbal Teas for Calm and Uplifted Emotions

1. Lemon Balm Emotional Reset Tea

- Brew 1 tablespoon dried lemon balm leaves in 1 cup hot water for 10 minutes.
- Sip to calm anxious thoughts and promote mental clarity.

2. Chamomile and Rose Petal Heart-Soothing Tea

- Steep 1 teaspoon dried chamomile and 1 teaspoon dried rose petals in hot water.
- Drink to ease emotional tension and open the heart.

3. **Passionflower Anti-Anxiety Tea**

   - Brew 1 teaspoon dried passionflower in 1 cup boiling water for 10 minutes.
   - Sip when feeling overwhelmed to calm the mind and soothe nervous energy.

4. **Holy Basil (Tulsi) Adaptogenic Tea**

   - Steep 1 teaspoon dried tulsi in 1 cup hot water for 10 minutes.
   - Drink to balance cortisol levels and reduce the physical effects of stress.

5. **Lavender and Lemon Zest Relaxation Tea**

   - Brew 1 teaspoon dried lavender flowers with a pinch of lemon zest.
   - Drink to relax after a busy day and prepare for restful sleep.

6. **Skullcap and Peppermint Nerve-Soothing Tea**

   - Combine 1 teaspoon dried skullcap with 1 teaspoon dried peppermint.
   - Steep in hot water for 10 minutes to relieve nervous tension and headaches.

7. **Ginger and Orange Sunshine Tea**

   - Simmer 1 teaspoon grated ginger with fresh orange peel in water for 5 minutes.
   - Sip to uplift your mood and energize your spirit.

8. **Oat Straw and Lavender Nervous System Tea**

- Brew 1 tablespoon dried oat straw with 1 teaspoon lavender flowers.
- Drink to nourish your nervous system and ease stress.

9. Rosehip and Hibiscus Mood Boost Tea

- Steep 1 teaspoon dried rosehips with 1 teaspoon dried hibiscus in hot water.
- Drink for a boost of vitamin C and to brighten your emotional outlook.

10. Raspberry Leaf and Chamomile Restorative Tea

- Brew 1 teaspoon dried raspberry leaf with 1 teaspoon chamomile.
- Sip to restore emotional balance and soothe frayed nerves.

Herbal Tinctures and Tonics for Emotional Balance

11. Ashwagandha Daily Resilience Tonic

- Take 1 dropper of ashwagandha tincture in water daily.
- Helps balance stress hormones and improve emotional stability.

12. Valerian Root Calm Tincture

- Use 1 dropper of valerian tincture in the evening to relax and unwind after a long day.

13. Lemon Balm and Holy Basil Emotional Relief Tonic

- Combine lemon balm and tulsi tinctures and take 1 dropper

when feeling overwhelmed.

- Helps soothe the mind and restore calm.

14. St. John's Wort Mood-Boosting Tincture

- Take 1 dropper of St. John's Wort tincture in the morning to lift your mood naturally.

15. Skullcap Nervine Tonic

- Take 1 dropper of skullcap tincture to calm frazzled nerves and emotional tension.

16. Rose Petal Uplift Tincture

- Steep fresh rose petals in vodka for 4 weeks, strain, and take 1 dropper to open your heart and promote joy.

17. Milky Oat Stress Recovery Tincture

- Take 1 dropper of milky oat tincture daily to repair an overworked nervous system.

18. Passionflower Sleep Aid Tonic

- Use 1 dropper of passionflower tincture before bed to calm racing thoughts and promote restful sleep.

19. Lavender and Lemon Balm Relaxation Blend

- Combine tinctures of lavender and lemon balm.

- Take 1 dropper to relieve tension and quiet the mind.

20. Chamomile and Honey Stress Tonic

- Mix 1 teaspoon chamomile tincture with 1 teaspoon raw honey.

- Stir into warm water and sip to ease emotional distress.

Mindfulness and Aromatherapy for Inner Peace

21. Frankincense and Myrrh Meditation Blend

- Add 3 drops frankincense oil and 2 drops myrrh oil to a diffuser.
- Use during meditation to ground your emotions and connect with your spirit.

22. Lavender and Orange Emotional Balance Mist

- Mix 1/4 cup distilled water with 5 drops lavender oil and 3 drops orange oil in a spray bottle.
- Mist the air around you to uplift your mood and promote calm.

23. Sandalwood and Patchouli Grounding Blend

- Add 3 drops sandalwood oil and 3 drops patchouli oil to a diffuser.
- Use to feel anchored and emotionally secure.

24. Rose and Geranium Heart-Opening Blend

- Combine 3 drops rose oil and 3 drops geranium oil in a diffuser.
- Use to release emotional tension and encourage self-love.

25. Lemon and Peppermint Focus Mist

- Mix 1/4 cup distilled water with 3 drops lemon oil and 3

drops peppermint oil.

- Mist your workspace to clear mental fog and uplift your spirits.

26. Mugwort Dream Pillow

- Fill a small fabric pouch with dried mugwort and lavender.
- Place under your pillow to encourage restful sleep and vivid dreams.

27. Chamomile and Lavender Bedtime Ritual Spray

- Combine 10 drops each of chamomile and lavender essential oil with 1/4 cup distilled water in a spray bottle.
- Mist your bedroom to create a calming sleep environment.

28. Sage and Cedar Clearing Ritual

- Burn sage and cedar together to clear your personal energy field.
- Use when feeling emotionally stuck or overwhelmed.

29. Mint and Basil Energizing Steam

- Add fresh mint and basil leaves to a bowl of hot water.
- Inhale deeply to energize your mind and refresh your mood.

30. Lemon Balm and Eucalyptus Morning Grounding Spray

- Mix lemon balm tincture with distilled water and 3 drops eucalyptus oil in a spray bottle.
- Mist around your space each morning to set a calm and focused tone for the day.

7.3 SPIRITUAL GROWTH

Spiritual growth is a deeply personal journey that involves self-reflection, mindfulness, and connecting with something greater than yourself. Herbs have long been used to support spiritual practices, whether through rituals, meditation, dreamwork, or energy clearing. Their grounding, heart-opening, and clarifying properties can help you align your inner self with your outer world, deepen your sense of purpose, and enhance your spiritual connection.

In this chapter, we'll explore herbal remedies that can aid in spiritual growth. From teas that enhance intuition to smudging rituals and dream-enhancing tools, these remedies will empower your journey inward and outward.

Herbal Teas and Tonics for Spiritual Connection

1. Mugwort Intuition Tea

- Steep 1 teaspoon dried mugwort in hot water for 5–10 minutes.
- Sip before meditation, journaling, or dreamwork to enhance intuition and inner vision.

2. Holy Basil (Tulsi) Grounding Tea

- Brew 1 teaspoon dried tulsi leaves in 1 cup hot water.
- Sip to center your spirit and prepare your mind for reflection or spiritual practices.

3. Blue Lotus Flower Meditation Tea

- Steep 1 tablespoon dried blue lotus petals in hot water for 10 minutes.
- Drink to promote relaxation, heightened awareness, and spiritual connection.

4. Rose and Lavender Heart-Opening Tea

- Brew 1 teaspoon dried rose petals with 1 teaspoon dried lavender flowers.
- Drink to open your heart to love, forgiveness, and emotional release.

5. Sage and Mint Clarity Tea

- Combine 1 teaspoon dried sage and 1 teaspoon dried peppermint in hot water.
- Sip to clear mental fog and align your thoughts with your intentions.

6. Chamomile and Lemon Balm Spiritual Calm Tea

- Brew 1 teaspoon each of dried chamomile and lemon balm.
- Sip before prayer or meditation to calm the mind and promote spiritual peace.

7. Hibiscus and Cinnamon Elevation Tea

- Brew 1 teaspoon dried hibiscus flowers with a pinch of cinnamon.
- Drink to uplift your spirit and align with higher vibrational energy.

8. Nettle and Rosemary Strength Tea

- Steep 1 tablespoon dried nettle with 1 teaspoon dried rosemary.
- Drink to ground your energy and build inner strength during challenging spiritual work.

9. Passionflower Dream Tea

- Brew 1 teaspoon dried passionflower in hot water for 10 minutes.
- Sip to relax before bed and invite spiritually meaningful dreams.

10. Ginger and Turmeric Awareness Tonic

- Simmer 1 teaspoon grated ginger and 1/2 teaspoon turmeric in water.
- Drink to promote clarity, mindfulness, and energy for your spiritual practices.

Herbal Tools and Rituals for Spiritual Practices

11. White Sage Smudge Stick for Energy Clearing

- Burn a bundle of dried white sage and use the smoke to cleanse your space.
- Ideal for clearing negative energy before meditation or rituals.

12. Palo Santo Spiritual Activation

- Light a stick of Palo Santo and allow its fragrant smoke to fill your space.
- Use to create a sacred atmosphere for reflection or spiritual

work.

13. Lavender and Rose Quartz Meditation Pouch

- Fill a small fabric pouch with dried lavender and a rose quartz crystal.
- Hold it during meditation to enhance emotional healing and love energy.

14. Mugwort and Bay Leaf Dream Pillow

- Fill a small pillow with dried mugwort and bay leaves.
- Place under your pillow to enhance dreams and connect with your subconscious.

15. Frankincense and Myrrh Cleansing Ritual

- Burn frankincense and myrrh resin on charcoal to purify your space.
- Use during spiritual ceremonies or when setting intentions.

16. Cedar and Rosemary Protection Bundle

- Tie together dried cedar and rosemary, and hang it near your entryway.
- Use to protect your space from negative energies.

17. Basil and Mint Abundance Ritual Spray

- Infuse fresh basil and mint leaves in water for 24 hours, then strain into a spray bottle.
- Spray your space to invite prosperity and positivity.

18. Rose Petal Offering Ritual

- Scatter dried rose petals around a sacred space or altar.
- Use as a symbolic offering of love, gratitude, or intention.

19. Lavender and Sage Aura Cleanse

- Burn a combination of dried lavender and sage.
- Walk through the smoke to cleanse your aura and refresh your spiritual energy.

20. Sandalwood and Cinnamon Sacred Space Mist

- Mix 1/4 cup distilled water with 3 drops sandalwood oil and 3 drops cinnamon oil.
- Mist your altar or sacred space before prayer or spiritual work.

Herbs for Meditation, Dreamwork, and Clarity

21. Blue Lotus Flower Meditation Oil

- Infuse dried blue lotus flowers in jojoba oil for 4 weeks.
- Use a few drops on your temples before meditation to heighten awareness.

22. Mugwort and Lavender Third Eye Steam

- Add dried mugwort and lavender to a bowl of steaming water.
- Cover your head with a towel and breathe deeply to awaken intuition and cleanse your third eye.

23. Peppermint and Eucalyptus Clarity Inhalation

- Add fresh peppermint and eucalyptus leaves to a bowl of hot water.
- Inhale deeply to clear your mind and sharpen focus.

24. Rosemary Memory Boost Diffuser Blend

- Add 3 drops rosemary oil and 2 drops lemon oil to a diffuser.
- Use to enhance memory, focus, and clarity during reflection or spiritual study.

25. Lavender and Mugwort Dream Bath

- Brew 1 tablespoon each of dried lavender and mugwort, strain, and add to your bath.
- Use to relax your body and invite meaningful dreams.

26. Yarrow Spiritual Strength Tea

- Brew 1 teaspoon dried yarrow in hot water.
- Drink to build courage and protect your energy during intense spiritual work.

27. Sage and Frankincense Third Eye Ritual Oil

- Infuse sage and frankincense resin in olive oil for 4 weeks.
- Apply a small amount to your third eye (center of the forehead) before meditation.

28. Lavender and Basil Focus Candle

- Sprinkle dried lavender and basil around the base of a white candle.
- Light during meditation or journaling to promote focus and

spiritual clarity.

29. Eucalyptus and Rosemary Shower Bundle

- Hang fresh eucalyptus and rosemary in your shower.
- The steam releases their energizing and cleansing aroma, perfect before meditation.

30. Rose and Hibiscus Altar Water

- Brew dried rose petals and hibiscus, then strain into a small bowl.
- Use this water on your altar as an offering or for cleansing spiritual tools.

PART 8: BEYOND THE BASICS

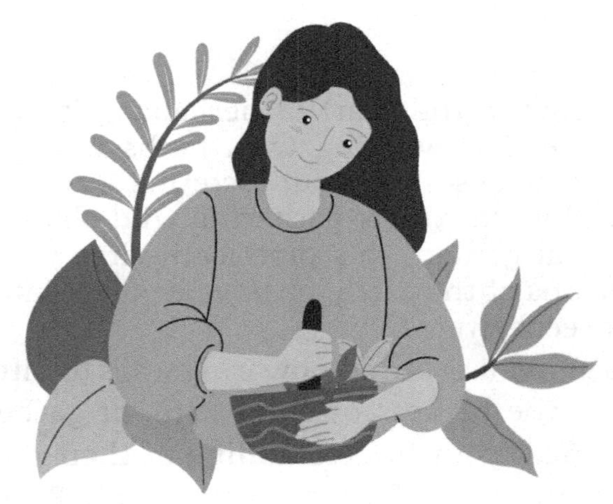

8.1 FORAGING AND GROWING YOUR OWN HERBS

As we come to the heart of herbalism, it's important to recognize that working with herbs is more than just using remedies—it's about fostering a deep relationship with nature. Whether you're gathering wild plants or growing your own herbal garden, this practice invites you to connect with the rhythms of the earth, observe its abundance, and care for its delicate ecosystems.

Foraging and gardening are empowering ways to integrate herbs into your life. The process of cultivating or gathering plants not only enhances your understanding of their properties but also deepens your respect for the natural world. Ethical foraging teaches us to take only what we need and to honor the environments that nurture these plants, while gardening gives us the opportunity to create sustainable, healing spaces right in our own backyards.

This chapter is a guide to responsibly and thoughtfully foraging wild herbs and cultivating your own herbal garden. It's about building a relationship with the earth that nurtures not only the plants but also your spirit. Let's explore how to ethically gather and grow herbs while being stewards of the land.

Ethical Foraging: Gathering Herbs in Harmony with Nature

Foraging allows you to discover herbs growing naturally in the wild, but it's important to gather responsibly to protect ecosystems and ensure the survival of plant populations for future generations. Here are tips to forage ethically:

1. Know the Laws and Permissions

- Always check local laws about foraging on public or private land. Some areas may have restrictions to protect plants and wildlife.

2. Identify Plants Correctly

- Learn to properly identify herbs before harvesting. Use field guides, attend foraging workshops, or work with experienced herbalists to ensure you're gathering the right plant. Mistakes can be dangerous.

3. Harvest Responsibly

- Follow the "1 in 5 rule": never take more than 20% of a plant population in a given area. Leave enough for wildlife and to ensure the plants can reproduce.
- Avoid foraging rare or endangered species. Instead, admire them and let them thrive in their natural habitat.

4. Harvest at the Right Time

- Gather plants when they are at their peak potency. For example:
    - **Leaves**: Early in the growing season.
    - **Flowers**: Just as they are blooming.
    - **Roots**: In late fall, after the plant has stored energy in its roots.

5. Protect the Habitat

- Avoid damaging the environment while foraging. Be gentle with roots, stems, and surrounding plants.
- Do not pull up entire plants unless absolutely necessary; focus on harvesting parts like leaves, flowers, or seeds.

6. Be Aware of Pollution

- Avoid foraging near roads, industrial areas, or places where herbicides or pesticides may have been used.

7. Give Thanks

- Treat foraging as a sacred practice. Offer gratitude to the plant and the earth for their gifts. Some herbalists leave small offerings, such as water or a spoken blessing, as a gesture of thanks.

Growing Your Own Herbs: Cultivating a Healing Garden

Starting your own herbal garden is one of the most rewarding ways to bring herbs into your life. Gardening allows you to work with fresh, vibrant plants, ensure sustainability, and create a peaceful space for reflection and connection to nature.

1. Start Small

- Begin with a few easy-to-grow herbs like basil, mint, calendula, and chamomile. These herbs thrive in most conditions and are useful for many remedies.

2. Choose the Right Location

- Select a spot with adequate sunlight (most herbs need at least 6 hours of direct sunlight daily).

- Ensure the soil is well-drained and rich in organic matter.

3. Use Containers for Limited Space

- If you don't have a garden, grow herbs in pots or containers on a balcony, windowsill, or patio. Herbs like thyme, oregano, and parsley do well in small spaces.

4. Companion Planting for Healthy Growth

- Pair herbs that support each other. For example:
    - Basil thrives next to tomatoes.
    - Lavender and rosemary benefit each other and repel pests.
    - Mint can grow aggressively, so plant it in its own container to prevent it from overtaking other herbs.

5. Harvest Regularly to Encourage Growth

- Regular pruning promotes healthy, bushy plants. For example, pinching the tips of basil plants encourages them to produce more leaves.

6. Use Organic Practices

- Avoid chemical fertilizers or pesticides. Instead, use compost to enrich the soil and natural pest repellents like neem oil or garlic spray.

7. Grow Perennials for Long-Term Use

- Plant perennial herbs like thyme, sage, and rosemary, which return year after year. This ensures a sustainable supply of fresh herbs.

8. Create a Pollinator-Friendly Garden

- Plant flowers like calendula, echinacea, and lavender to attract bees and butterflies. Pollinators play a vital role in the health of your garden and the environment.

9. Save Seeds for the Next Season

- Let some herbs like dill, coriander (cilantro), or basil flower and go to seed. Collect seeds to plant in the next growing season or to share with friends.

10. Make It a Healing Space

- Design your garden with intention. Add a bench, fountain, or pathway to create a peaceful retreat where you can connect with nature and reflect.

Harvesting and Preserving Your Herbs

Growing or foraging herbs is only the first step—you also need to know how to harvest and preserve them for long-term use while maintaining their potency.

1. Harvest in the Morning

- Collect herbs early in the day, after the dew has dried but before the sun becomes too intense. This is when their essential oils are most concentrated.

2. Dry Herbs Properly

- Tie small bundles of herbs and hang them upside down in a cool, dark, and well-ventilated area. Alternatively, use a dehydrator on the lowest setting.
- Ensure herbs are completely dry before storing to prevent mold.

3. Store Herbs Correctly

- Keep dried herbs in airtight containers away from direct sunlight and moisture. Use glass jars or tins for the best preservation.

4. Freeze Herbs for Freshness

- Chop fresh herbs and freeze them in ice cube trays with a bit of water or olive oil. This method preserves their flavor for cooking or remedies.

5. Make Herbal Infusions

- Steep fresh or dried herbs in vinegar, oil, or alcohol to create tinctures, infused oils, and vinegars. These can be stored for months and used for culinary or medicinal purposes.

6. Label and Rotate

- Label your herbs with the name and date of harvest. Use older batches first to ensure you're working with the freshest materials.

Final Thoughts

Foraging and growing your own herbs is a deeply fulfilling way to integrate herbalism into your life. It connects you with the land, teaches patience and care, and allows you to take an active role in your healing journey. By foraging ethically and gardening sustainably, you not only create a personal supply of fresh herbs but also nurture the earth that provides them.

In the next chapter, we'll explore Preserving and Storing Herbal Remedies, where we'll dive deeper into techniques for keeping your herbs fresh and potent for years to come. Let's continue!

8.2 PRESERVING AND STORING HERBAL REMEDIES

Once you've harvested or prepared your herbs, knowing how to store them properly is essential to maintain their potency and effectiveness. Herbs can lose their therapeutic properties when exposed to moisture, light, air, or heat, so taking care during the preservation and storage process ensures that their healing benefits are retained for months—or even years.

This chapter focuses on how to properly preserve herbal remedies, including drying, freezing, and creating long-lasting preparations like tinctures, oils, and syrups. By following these simple methods, you can extend the shelf life of your herbs and create a reliable apothecary for your health and wellness needs.

Why Proper Preservation Matters

Herbs are living materials that begin to lose their potency as soon as they're harvested. Over time, essential oils dissipate, flavors fade, and medicinal compounds degrade. Proper preservation methods can:

- Extend the shelf life of herbal remedies.
- Protect herbs from moisture, mold, and contamination.
- Ensure you're working with fresh, effective materials for teas, tinctures, and other remedies.
- Save money by minimizing waste and maximizing your

harvest.

Let's explore the best ways to preserve and store herbs for long-term use.

---

1. Drying Herbs for Long-Term Use

Drying is the most common way to preserve herbs. It removes moisture, which prevents mold and spoilage, while concentrating the flavor and medicinal properties of the plant.

Steps to Dry Herbs

1. **Harvest at the Right Time**:
   - Collect herbs in the morning, after dew has dried but before the sun becomes too strong.
   - For leaves, harvest before the plant flowers. For flowers, harvest when they are just blooming.
2. **Prepare for Drying**:
   - Gently shake off dirt or debris. Avoid washing unless absolutely necessary, as water can delay drying and encourage mold.
3. **Air-Drying (Best for Leaves, Flowers, and Stems)**:
   - Tie herbs into small bundles with twine or rubber bands.
   - Hang upside down in a cool, dark, and well-ventilated area.
   - Allow 1–2 weeks for herbs to dry completely. They should feel brittle to the touch.
4. **Dehydrator Drying**:

- Place herbs on dehydrator trays in a single layer.
- Set the dehydrator to its lowest setting (95–115°F).
- Check regularly and remove when herbs are completely dry.

5. **Oven Drying (For Faster Results)**:
   - Preheat your oven to its lowest setting (typically around 170°F).
   - Spread herbs on a baking sheet in a single layer.
   - Dry with the oven door slightly ajar to allow moisture to escape, and check frequently to avoid overheating.

---

2. Storing Dried Herbs

Once dried, herbs must be stored properly to prevent them from absorbing moisture or losing their potency.

Best Practices for Storage

- **Use Airtight Containers**: Store herbs in glass jars, tins, or tightly-sealed bags to protect them from air and moisture.
- **Keep Away from Light**: Light causes herbs to lose their color and potency. Use dark glass jars or store in a dark pantry.
- **Label Clearly**: Write the name of the herb and the date it was dried on the container. Rotate your stock to use older herbs first.
- **Check Periodically**: Inspect your herbs regularly for signs of mold, discoloration, or loss of aroma.

Shelf Life of Dried Herbs

- **Leaves and Flowers**: 1 year (aromatic herbs like mint or basil may lose potency sooner).

- **Roots and Bark**: 2–3 years (if stored properly).
- **Seeds**: Up to 3 years.

---

3. Freezing Herbs for Freshness

Freezing is another effective way to preserve herbs, especially for culinary use. Freezing preserves the flavor and medicinal properties of fresh herbs, though the texture may change after thawing.

Steps for Freezing Herbs

1. **Chop and Portion**:
   - Wash herbs thoroughly and pat dry.
   - Chop into small pieces and portion into ice cube trays.
2. **Freeze with Liquid**:
   - Fill each ice cube slot with herbs and cover with water, olive oil, or broth.
   - Freeze overnight, then transfer frozen cubes to a labeled freezer-safe bag or container.
3. **Store and Use**:
   - Frozen herbs can be added directly to soups, teas, or remedies as needed.

Best Herbs for Freezing

- Basil, parsley, mint, dill, chives, and cilantro freeze well.

---

4. Preserving Herbs in Oils and Vinegars

Infusing herbs into oils or vinegars is an excellent way to preserve their flavor and medicinal properties while creating versatile ingredients for remedies or cooking.

Herbal Infused Oils

- **Method**:
  - Fill a clean, dry jar halfway with fresh or dried herbs.
  - Cover completely with a carrier oil like olive oil or almond oil.
  - Seal the jar and let it infuse for 4–6 weeks in a cool, dark place, shaking occasionally.
  - Strain the oil through a fine sieve or cheesecloth and store in a dark glass bottle.
- **Shelf Life**:
  - Infused oils last 6–12 months if stored in a cool, dark place.

Herbal Vinegars

- **Method**:
  - Fill a jar halfway with fresh or dried herbs.
  - Cover completely with vinegar (apple cider vinegar is ideal).
  - Seal the jar and let it infuse for 2–4 weeks, shaking occasionally.
  - Strain and store in a glass bottle.
- **Shelf Life**:
  - Herbal vinegars last 6–12 months.

5. Herbal Syrups for Long-Term Use

Syrups combine the potency of herbal decoctions with the sweetness of honey or sugar to create long-lasting remedies for colds, coughs, and immune support.

How to Make Herbal Syrups

1. **Prepare a Decoction**:
   - Simmer herbs (like elderberries or licorice root) in water for 30–45 minutes to extract their medicinal properties.
2. **Strain and Sweeten**:
   - Strain the liquid and return to the pot. Add honey (or sugar) in a 2:1 ratio (two parts decoction to one part sweetener).
3. **Bottle and Store**:
   - Pour into sterilized glass bottles or jars.
   - Store in the refrigerator for up to 6 months.

6. Creating Herbal Powders

Herbal powders are convenient for teas, capsules, and smoothies.

Steps for Making Herbal Powders

1. **Dry Herbs Thoroughly**:
   - Ensure herbs are completely dry to prevent mold.
2. **Grind into Powder**:
   - Use a mortar and pestle, spice grinder, or blender to

grind herbs into a fine powder.

3. **Store Properly**:
    - Keep powders in airtight containers away from light and moisture.
    - Label with the name of the herb and date of preparation.

Shelf Life of Herbal Powders

- Up to 1 year if stored in ideal conditions.

Final Thoughts

Preserving and storing herbs properly allows you to build a robust home apothecary that supports your wellness year-round. Whether drying, freezing, or creating infused oils and syrups, these methods ensure that your remedies remain potent and effective. Treat your herbal remedies with care, and they'll reward you with their healing properties when you need them most.

8.3 SHARING HERBAL WISDOM

Sharing your herbal knowledge with others helps spread the beauty and healing power of plants. Whether it's through meaningful gifts, DIY workshops, or heartfelt conversations, teaching and giving herbal remedies can inspire others to reconnect with nature and their own well-being.
This chapter explores creative ways to gift herbal remedies and teach herbal practices to friends, family, and your community. From beautifully packaged teas and oils to DIY classes and herb kits, these ideas celebrate the joy of passing on herbal wisdom in meaningful, accessible ways.

Why Share Herbal Wisdom?

- **Connection**: Sharing herbal remedies fosters deeper connections with others. It's a gift of health, care, and intention.
- **Empowerment**: Teaching others about herbs empowers them to take control of their own well-being.
- **Tradition**: Herbalism is a practice that has been passed down for centuries. Sharing your knowledge keeps these traditions alive.
- **Community**: By gifting or teaching herbs, you help build a community that values natural health and sustainability.

Let's explore creative and meaningful ways to share herbal

wisdom through gifts and teaching.

---

1. Creative Ways to Gift Herbal Remedies

1. Handcrafted Herbal Tea Blends

- Mix dried herbs like chamomile, peppermint, and rose petals into a custom tea blend.
- Package in small glass jars or resealable pouches with handwritten labels and brewing instructions.
- Personalize each blend for the recipient, such as a calming bedtime tea or an energizing morning mix.

2. Herbal Bath Soaks

- Combine dried lavender, rose petals, and Epsom salts in a fabric sachet or jar.
- Add a few drops of essential oil for a luxurious scent.
- Include a note about the benefits of a soothing herbal bath.

3. DIY Herbal Infused Oils

- Infuse olive oil or almond oil with herbs like calendula, lavender, or rosemary.
- Bottle the infused oil in small, decorative jars with a tag that explains its uses (e.g., for massage, skincare, or cooking).

4. Herbal Syrups for Cold and Flu Season

- Create elderberry syrup or a ginger-honey elixir.
- Pour into sterilized glass bottles, and tie a ribbon with a recipe card or serving instructions.

5. Herbal Seed Kits

- Gather small packets of seeds for beginner-friendly herbs like basil, mint, and calendula.
- Place them in a box with planting instructions, a small pot, and soil pellets.
- Perfect for introducing someone to the joy of growing their own herbs.

6. Smudge Stick Bundles

- Create smudge bundles with dried sage, lavender, and rosemary tied with natural twine.
- Include a note explaining how to use smudge sticks for energy clearing or meditation.

7. Herbal Dream Pillows

- Sew or buy small fabric pouches and fill them with herbs like mugwort, lavender, and chamomile.
- Gift as a tool to promote restful sleep and dreamwork.

8. Aromatherapy Room Sprays

- Mix distilled water with essential oils like peppermint, lavender, or eucalyptus in a spray bottle.
- Add a label with instructions for misting rooms, linens, or pillows.

9. Herbal Baking Gifts

- Bake lavender shortbread cookies, rosemary bread, or mint brownies.
- Package with a note describing the herbs' health benefits.

10. Personalized Herbal Gift Baskets

- Create themed gift baskets such as "Relaxation" (lavender oil, chamomile tea, bath salts) or "Cold and Flu Relief" (elderberry syrup, ginger tea, eucalyptus steam blend).

---

2. Teaching Herbal Wisdom

1. Host a DIY Herbal Workshop

- Invite friends or community members to a workshop where they can make simple remedies like teas, tinctures, or bath salts.
- Provide all materials and a brief introduction to each herb.

2. Share Recipes and Guides

- Write out your favorite herbal recipes (like tea blends, tinctures, or salves) and share them as printed cards or a small booklet.
- Add notes about each herb's benefits and tips for preparation.

3. Create Online Tutorials

- Film a video or write a blog post demonstrating how to make an herbal remedy, such as a calming tea or a healing salve.
- Share it on social media or your own website to reach a wider audience.

4. Offer a Plant Walk or Foraging Class

- Take a small group on a guided nature walk to identify local herbs.

- Teach them how to forage ethically, identify plants, and use them in remedies.

5. Build Beginner Herb Kits

- Assemble kits with essential herbs like chamomile, peppermint, and calendula, along with instructions for making simple remedies.
- Include reusable tea bags or small jars to encourage experimentation.

6. Teach Herbal Gardening Basics

- Share tips on how to grow herbs in pots or gardens, especially beginner-friendly ones like basil, thyme, and parsley.
- Consider gifting cuttings or potted herbs as part of the lesson.

7. Lead a Meditation with Herbal Support

- Incorporate herbal teas or essential oils into a meditation or mindfulness session.
- For example, use lavender for relaxation or peppermint for focus.

8. Host a Tea Tasting Party

- Invite friends to sample different herbal teas.
- Provide information about each herb, its flavor, and its benefits.

9. Write a Beginner's Herbalism Guide

- Create a small booklet or PDF that introduces common herbs, their benefits, and how to use them.
- Share it digitally or as a printed handout.

10. Create a Community Herbal Library

- Collect books, guides, and field journals about herbalism and share them with your local community or friends.
- Encourage others to borrow, learn, and grow their knowledge.

---

3. Inspiring Others to Explore Herbalism

1. Share Stories and Experiences

- Talk about your own journey with herbs, including successes and challenges.
- Sharing personal stories makes herbalism approachable and inspiring.

2. Lead by Example

- Use herbal remedies in your daily life, and let others see how they support your well-being.
- Share a cup of herbal tea with a friend or use your own salves during conversations.

3. Create an Herbal Gratitude Circle

- Gather a group to share herbal remedies they've made, with each person explaining how the herb has helped them.
- Encourage sharing of knowledge and experiences.

4. Gift "Herbal Inspiration Notes"

- Write small notes with quotes, affirmations, or interesting herbal facts, and include them with your gifts.
- These can inspire curiosity and spark interest in herbs.

5. Collaborate with Local Groups

- Partner with community centers, schools, or wellness groups to teach or demonstrate simple herbal remedies.
- Consider focusing on accessible and affordable herbs like chamomile, mint, and lemon balm.

6. Organize a Seed Exchange

- Host a gathering where participants can trade herb seeds, cuttings, or small plants.
- Share tips on growing each herb and encourage discussions about their uses.

7. Celebrate the Seasons with Herbs

- Host seasonal events, like spring planting workshops or autumn herb harvesting gatherings.
- Focus on herbs that are in season and how to use them.

8. Share Herbal Crafts

- Teach creative uses for herbs, such as making wreaths, sachets, or natural dyes.
- These projects can show how herbs go beyond remedies and into art and beauty.

9. Create Herbal Challenges

- Encourage friends or community members to try a new herb every week.
- Share recipes and experiences, making it a fun, engaging way to learn together.

10. Offer Kindness with Herbs

- Share herbal remedies with someone who may need them —a friend recovering from illness, a tired parent, or a busy colleague.
- A small jar of tea or a soothing balm can make a meaningful difference in their day.

Final Thoughts

Sharing herbal wisdom is a way of giving back—to your community, your loved ones, and the earth itself. Whether you're crafting gifts, teaching classes, or simply sharing a cup of tea, these small acts of generosity can inspire curiosity, healing, and connection. Herbalism is a gift that grows, strengthening bonds and bringing the natural world into more lives.

As you continue your herbal journey, remember that every remedy you give, every lesson you teach, and every plant you share spreads the wisdom of nature. By sharing herbalism, you plant seeds of knowledge and care that will bloom far beyond what you can see.

8.4 THE JOURNEY OF A HOME HERBALIST

Congratulations, my friend—you've come so far on your journey into the world of herbs! Whether you started this book with just a passing curiosity or a burning desire to transform your life with nature's gifts, you've made incredible progress. You've explored the healing power of herbs, created remedies, learned how to grow and forage, and even discovered ways to share your wisdom with others. That's something to celebrate!

Take a moment to reflect on all you've accomplished. You've tapped into traditions that are as old as humanity itself. You've reclaimed knowledge that was once passed down through families and communities—a way of healing that connects us to the earth, to ourselves, and to each other.

This chapter is about honoring your growth, acknowledging the beauty of this journey, and looking ahead to what's next. Herbalism isn't something you "finish"—it's a lifelong practice of learning, growing, and connecting with the natural world. So let's talk about where you've been, what you've learned, and how you can keep growing as a home herbalist.

Celebrate Your Progress

When you began, you may have felt unsure about your ability to work with herbs. Maybe you wondered if you'd be able to tell chamomile from calendula, or if you'd ever get the hang of making a tincture or drying herbs. But here you are—you've done it! You've turned curiosity into action, and action into knowledge.

Take pride in every step of the journey you've taken so far:

- The first time you brewed a cup of herbal tea and felt its calming effects.
- The joy of harvesting your own herbs or foraging responsibly in nature.
- The sense of accomplishment when you blended your first salve, tincture, or bath soak.
- The moment you shared an herbal remedy with a loved one and saw their gratitude.

Each small victory is a milestone. And each remedy you've made, herb you've worked with, or lesson you've learned is part of a much bigger story—your story as a home herbalist.

Remember, herbalism isn't about perfection. It's about presence. It's about building a relationship with plants, experimenting, and learning as you go. Every herbalist starts as a beginner, and even the most experienced herbalists are still learning. You're exactly where you're meant to be.

What's Next on Your Herbal Journey?

As you celebrate how far you've come, it's natural to wonder, "What's next?" The beauty of herbalism is that there's always more to explore. Here are a few ideas to inspire your next steps:

1. Deepen Your Knowledge

- **Focus on a Few Herbs**: Choose three or four herbs to get to know on a deeper level. Study their properties, experiment with different preparations, and observe how they work with your body.

- **Learn from the Masters**: Dive into herbal books, attend workshops, or study with experienced herbalists. There's so much wisdom out there waiting to be discovered.
- **Explore Traditional Practices**: Learn about the herbal traditions of different cultures, such as Traditional Chinese Medicine, Ayurveda, or Indigenous herbalism.

2. Expand Your Skills

- **Grow Your Apothecary**: Start building a more comprehensive collection of dried herbs, tinctures, oils, and syrups.
- **Try Advanced Preparations**: Experiment with more complex remedies like herbal wines, oxymels (vinegar-honey preparations), or even natural skincare products.
- **Preserve the Harvest**: Learn new ways to preserve your herbs, such as making powders, infused honeys, or herbal vinegars.

3. Connect with Nature

- **Forage More Confidently**: Practice identifying and harvesting wild herbs ethically and respectfully.
- **Grow Your Garden**: Expand your herb garden or start one if you haven't already. Include perennial herbs that will return year after year, like sage, thyme, and echinacea.
- **Journal with Nature**: Spend quiet moments observing the plants around you. Write about their growth, their cycles, and the ways they influence you.

4. Share Your Herbal Wisdom

- **Teach Others**: Share your knowledge with friends, family, or your community. Host a workshop, write a blog, or create simple DIY kits to introduce others to herbalism.
- **Make Gifts**: Continue creating herbal gifts for loved ones—tea blends, infused oils, bath soaks, or dream pillows.
- **Build Your Herbal Network**: Connect with other herbalists, join local foraging or gardening groups, or participate in online herbal communities.

5. **Trust Your Intuition**

- The more you work with herbs, the more you'll develop a sense of what your body and spirit need. Trust that intuition. It's part of the wisdom you're cultivating as a home herbalist.

Challenges Are Part of the Journey

Every herbalist faces challenges along the way. Maybe you overharvested a plant by mistake or misidentified an herb. Maybe you struggled with a remedy that didn't turn out the way you'd hoped. That's okay! Mistakes are opportunities to learn.

Herbalism is about patience and humility. Plants remind us to slow down, observe, and respect the natural world. As you continue your journey, remember to embrace the lessons in every challenge.

The Gift of Herbalism

Herbalism is more than just a practice—it's a gift. It connects you to the earth, to your ancestors, and to the wisdom of countless generations who turned to plants for healing. It reminds us that we are part of nature, not separate from it, and that healing comes from living in harmony with the world around us.

As you continue on this path, you'll not only deepen your relationship with plants but also with yourself. You'll notice the ways herbs help you slow down, listen, and care for your body, mind, and spirit. And you'll carry that wisdom with you into every part of your life.

A Final Reflection

Take a moment now to reflect on the journey you've started. Picture yourself a year from now—how will your herbal practice have grown? Will you be tending a thriving garden, teaching a class, or simply sitting with a cup of homemade tea, marveling at how far you've come?

Whatever path you take, trust that it will be uniquely yours. There is no "right" way to be an herbalist. There is only your way—your curiosity, your creativity, and your connection to the plants.

Thank you for letting this book guide you as you took your first steps into herbalism. I hope it's been as inspiring for you as it was for me to share these words with you. May you continue to grow, to learn, and to heal with the wisdom of nature.

Your Next Steps

- Revisit the chapters in this book whenever you need a refresher or inspiration.
- Experiment with new remedies, recipes, and techniques.
- Stay curious, and don't be afraid to ask questions or explore new ideas.

Above all, remember that herbalism is a lifelong journey. There will always be more to learn, more to share, and more ways to grow.

Cheers to your journey as a home herbalist—may it bring you joy, health, and a deep sense of connection to the earth and all its wonders.

Here's to you and the world of herbs—happy growing, crafting, and healing ;)

APPENDICES

HERBAL QUICK REFERENCE GUIDE

This quick reference guide is designed to help you find the right herbs at a glance. Whether you're crafting a remedy, making a tea, or looking for natural support for a specific issue, this cheat sheet offers a concise overview of popular herbs and their primary uses. Each herb is paired with its key properties and a few quick tips for how to use it.

Adaptogens *(Herbs that help the body adapt to stress and support overall balance)*

Ashwagandha

- **Key Uses**: Reduces stress, supports adrenal health, promotes restful sleep.
- **How to Use**: Add to teas, smoothies, or make a daily tincture.
- **Tip**: Great for long-term use to rebuild strength after burnout.

Holy Basil (Tulsi)

- **Key Uses**: Balances cortisol, calms the mind, boosts energy.
- **How to Use**: Brew as a tea for relaxation and focus.
- **Tip**: Ideal for daily use during stressful times.

Rhodiola

- **Key Uses**: Increases energy, reduces fatigue, improves mental focus.
- **How to Use**: Take as a tincture or in capsules.
- **Tip**: Use for short bursts of energy; best taken in the morning.

Maca

- **Key Uses**: Balances hormones, boosts energy and stamina.
- **How to Use**: Add to smoothies or mix into warm drinks.
- **Tip**: Great for pre-workout energy and hormonal support.

Calming and Nervine Herbs *(Herbs that calm the nervous system and reduce stress)*

Chamomile

- **Key Uses**: Calms anxiety, aids sleep, soothes digestion.
- **How to Use**: Brew as a tea or use in a calming bath soak.
- **Tip**: Perfect for winding down at bedtime.

Lavender

- **Key Uses**: Relieves tension, supports relaxation, soothes headaches.
- **How to Use**: Use in aromatherapy, teas, or bath salts.
- **Tip**: Place a sachet under your pillow for better sleep.

Lemon Balm

- **Key Uses**: Eases anxiety, boosts mood, promotes clarity.
- **How to Use**: Drink as a tea or use in a tincture.
- **Tip**: Excellent for uplifting spirits during emotional overwhelm.

Passionflower

- **Key Uses**: Reduces anxiety, calms racing thoughts, aids sleep.
- **How to Use**: Brew as a tea or use as a tincture.
- **Tip**: Take before bed to quiet the mind and promote deep sleep.

Immune Boosters *(Herbs that strengthen the immune system and fight infections)*

Elderberry

- **Key Uses**: Prevents and treats colds and flu, antiviral properties.
- **How to Use**: Make syrup, tea, or gummies.
- **Tip**: Take at the first sign of illness to shorten recovery time.

Echinacea

- **Key Uses**: Stimulates immune response, fights colds and infections.
- **How to Use**: Brew as tea or use as a tincture.
- **Tip**: Best used during the first few days of illness.

Astragalus

- **Key Uses**: Builds long-term immunity, supports overall vitality.
- **How to Use**: Simmer in soups or brew as tea.
- **Tip**: Use consistently during cold and flu season for prevention.

Garlic

- **Key Uses**: Antiviral, antibacterial, strengthens the immune system.
- **How to Use**: Eat raw, infuse in honey, or make garlic vinegar.
- **Tip**: Crush garlic and let it sit for 10 minutes before use to activate its medicinal properties.

Digestive Support *(Herbs that soothe digestion and improve gut health)*

Peppermint

- **Key Uses**: Relieves bloating, nausea, and indigestion.
- **How to Use**: Brew as tea or use in a steam inhalation.
- **Tip**: Great for calming upset stomachs after meals.

Ginger

- **Key Uses**: Eases nausea, supports digestion, reduces inflammation.
- **How to Use**: Make ginger tea, add to soups, or chew fresh slices.

- **Tip**: Sip ginger tea during travel to combat motion sickness.

Fennel

- **Key Uses**: Reduces gas, bloating, and colic.
- **How to Use**: Brew fennel seeds as tea or chew after meals.
- **Tip**: Safe and gentle for children experiencing digestive discomfort.

Slippery Elm

- **Key Uses**: Soothes the stomach lining, helps with acid reflux.
- **How to Use**: Make a paste with warm water and slippery elm powder.
- **Tip**: Drink before meals to coat and protect the stomach.

Pain and Inflammation Relief *(Herbs that ease pain and reduce inflammation)*

Turmeric

- **Key Uses**: Anti-inflammatory, supports joint health, relieves pain.
- **How to Use**: Add to golden milk, smoothies, or capsules.
- **Tip**: Combine with black pepper to enhance absorption.

Willow Bark

- **Key Uses**: Natural pain reliever, reduces headaches and muscle pain.
- **How to Use**: Brew as a tea or use in tinctures.

- **Tip**: Known as "nature's aspirin."

Arnica

- **Key Uses**: Reduces swelling, soothes bruises and sore muscles (external use only).
- **How to Use**: Apply as a salve or infused oil to the affected area.
- **Tip**: Keep an arnica salve handy for post-workout soreness.

Devil's Claw

- **Key Uses**: Eases joint pain, reduces inflammation, supports arthritis relief.
- **How to Use**: Take as a tincture or capsule.
- **Tip**: Particularly effective for chronic pain.

Skin Healing Herbs *(Herbs that treat cuts, burns, rashes, and other skin conditions)*

Calendula

- **Key Uses**: Heals wounds, reduces inflammation, soothes dry skin.
- **How to Use**: Make an infused oil or salve.
- **Tip**: Perfect for diaper rash and other sensitive skin issues.

Aloe Vera

- **Key Uses**: Soothes burns, hydrates skin, reduces irritation.
- **How to Use**: Apply fresh gel directly to burns or inflamed areas.

- **Tip**: Keep an aloe vera plant in your home for quick use.

Plantain

- **Key Uses**: Heals cuts, insect bites, and rashes; draws out toxins.
- **How to Use**: Crush fresh leaves into a poultice and apply to skin.
- **Tip**: Excellent for soothing itchy bug bites.

Witch Hazel

- **Key Uses**: Reduces inflammation, tightens skin, treats acne.
- **How to Use**: Apply as a toner or compress.
- **Tip**: Keep a bottle of witch hazel in your first-aid kit for quick use.

Herbs for Emotional Wellness *(Herbs that calm, uplift, and restore emotional balance)*

St. John's Wort

- **Key Uses**: Eases mild depression, supports emotional balance.
- **How to Use**: Take as a tincture or capsule.
- **Tip**: Avoid excessive sun exposure while using St. John's Wort, as it can increase sensitivity.

Rose Petals

- **Key Uses**: Opens the heart, promotes self-love, calms the spirit.

- **How to Use**: Brew as a tea or use in bath salts.
- **Tip**: Add dried rose petals to sachets for a comforting scent.

Skullcap

- **Key Uses**: Soothes frazzled nerves, calms anxiety, eases emotional overload.
- **How to Use**: Brew as tea or take as a tincture.
- **Tip**: Ideal for moments of high stress or emotional exhaustion.

Hibiscus

- **Key Uses**: Uplifts mood, supports heart health, provides antioxidants.
- **How to Use**: Brew as tea, hot or iced.
- **Tip**: Its vibrant red color makes it a cheerful and refreshing tea option.

This cheat sheet is designed to be a quick resource as you explore herbal remedies. Whether you're brewing a tea, making a salve, or crafting a tincture, let these herbs inspire you to connect with nature's healing gifts. Keep experimenting, learning, and trusting the wisdom of the plants!

GLOSSARY

A

- **Adaptogens**: Herbs that help the body adapt to stress, regulate cortisol levels, and restore balance in the body. Examples include ashwagandha, tulsi, and rhodiola.
- **Aromatherapy**: The use of essential oils derived from plants to support emotional, physical, and spiritual well-being through inhalation or topical application.
- **Anti-inflammatory**: Herbs or substances that reduce inflammation in the body. Examples include turmeric, ginger, and calendula.
- **Antimicrobial**: Herbs that kill or inhibit the growth of harmful microorganisms, such as bacteria, viruses, or fungi. Examples include garlic, thyme, and tea tree.
- **Antioxidants**: Compounds that protect cells from damage caused by free radicals. Found in herbs like hibiscus, green tea, and rosehips.
- **Antispasmodic**: Herbs that relax muscle spasms or cramps. Examples include chamomile, cramp bark, and peppermint.
- **Astringent**: Herbs that tighten tissues, reduce bleeding, or tone the skin. Examples include witch hazel, yarrow, and rose.

B

- **Bitters**: Herbs that stimulate digestion by activating bitter receptors in the tongue and digestive tract. Examples include dandelion root, gentian, and wormwood.
- **Botanical**: Refers to plants or plant-based products used for medicinal, therapeutic, or cosmetic purposes.

C

- **Calendula**: A gentle herb with anti-inflammatory and skin-healing properties, often used in salves and creams for cuts, burns, and rashes.
- **Carrier Oil**: A neutral oil, such as olive, almond, or coconut oil, used to dilute essential oils or infuse herbs for topical application.
- **Compress**: A cloth soaked in an herbal infusion or decoction, applied externally to soothe injuries, inflammation, or pain.
- **Cold Infusion**: A method of extracting herbal properties by soaking herbs in cold water for an extended period, often used for mucilaginous herbs like marshmallow root.
- **Cooling Herbs**: Herbs that reduce heat in the body and calm inflammation. Examples include peppermint, lemon balm, and cucumber.
- **Cramp Bark**: An herb known for its ability to relax uterine and muscle cramps.

D

- **Decoction**: A method of extracting medicinal properties by simmering tough plant materials like roots, bark, or seeds in water for an extended period.

- **Detoxification (Detox)**: The process of removing toxins from the body using herbs that support the liver, kidneys, and lymphatic system. Examples include dandelion, burdock, and nettle.
- **Distillation**: The process of extracting essential oils or hydrosols from plants by steaming and condensing the plant's aromatic compounds.
- **Drying Herbs**: The process of preserving herbs by removing their moisture to prevent spoilage and mold.

E

- **Elderberry**: A powerful immune-boosting herb often used in syrups to prevent and treat colds and flu.
- **Electrolytes**: Minerals like potassium, magnesium, and sodium that help regulate hydration and body function. Herbal electrolyte drinks can include ingredients like coconut water, nettle, and chia seeds.
- **Essential Oils**: Highly concentrated plant oils extracted through distillation, used in aromatherapy and topical applications. Examples include lavender, eucalyptus, and tea tree.
- **Ethical Foraging**: The practice of gathering wild plants responsibly to ensure the environment and plant populations remain healthy and sustainable.

F

- **Flower Essence**: A liquid infusion made by steeping flowers in water under sunlight, believed to carry the energetic properties of the plant to support emotional or spiritual well-being.

- **Foraging**: The act of gathering herbs, plants, or mushrooms in the wild for culinary, medicinal, or therapeutic use.

H

- **Harvesting**: The process of gathering herbs at the appropriate time to maximize their potency and effectiveness.

- **Healing Salve**: A balm made by infusing herbs into a carrier oil, thickened with beeswax, and used to heal cuts, burns, and rashes.

- **Herbal Actions**: The therapeutic effects of herbs on the body, such as being anti-inflammatory, adaptogenic, or antimicrobial.

- **Hydrosol**: A byproduct of essential oil distillation, often called "flower water," used for skincare and therapeutic purposes.

I

- **Infusion**: A method of extracting herbal properties by steeping herbs in hot water, similar to making tea.

- **Infused Oils**: Carrier oils infused with herbs to extract their medicinal properties for topical use. Examples include calendula oil and arnica oil.

L

- **Lymphatic System**: A network in the body that helps remove waste and toxins. Herbs like calendula and cleavers support lymphatic drainage and cleansing.

M

- **Medicinal Herbs**: Plants used to prevent or treat ailments, promote wellness, or support the body's natural healing processes. Examples include ginger, garlic, and echinacea.
- **Moistening Herbs**: Herbs that restore moisture and soothe dryness in the body. Examples include marshmallow root and slippery elm.
- **Mucilage**: A gel-like substance in some herbs that soothes and coats mucous membranes. Found in plants like marshmallow root and slippery elm.
- **Mugwort**: An herb known for enhancing dreams, calming anxiety, and supporting digestive health.

O

- **Oxymel**: A herbal preparation made by infusing herbs in a mixture of honey and vinegar, often used for colds, coughs, and digestion.

P

- **Perennials**: Herbs that grow back year after year, such as rosemary, thyme, and mint.
- **Poultice**: A paste made from fresh or dried herbs that is applied directly to the skin to treat wounds, inflammation, or pain.
- **Preservation**: Methods used to store herbs and remedies for long-term use, such as drying, freezing, or creating tinctures and oils.

S

- **Smudging**: The practice of burning herbs like sage, cedar, or palo santo to clear negative energy or purify a space.
- **Solar Infusion**: A method of infusing herbs into oil or water using sunlight to gently extract their properties.
- **Strainer**: A tool used to separate herbs from liquid after brewing or infusing. Fine mesh strainers or cheesecloth work well.
- **Syrup**: A sweetened herbal preparation made by combining a concentrated decoction with honey or sugar, often used for colds and flu.

T

- **Tincture**: A concentrated herbal extract made by steeping herbs in alcohol or glycerin. Used as a long-lasting remedy for various ailments.
- **Tonics**: Herbal preparations that strengthen and restore the body's systems over time. Examples include nettle tea for vitality or ashwagandha for stress relief.
- **Topical Application**: Using herbs externally on the skin in forms such as salves, poultices, or infused oils.

W

- **Wildcrafting**: The practice of harvesting wild plants for medicinal or culinary use in a sustainable and respectful manner.
- **Warming Herbs**: Herbs that increase circulation, promote warmth in the body, and support digestion. Examples include ginger, cinnamon, and cayenne.

Y

- **Yarrow**: A versatile herb used for wound healing, reducing fevers, and toning the skin.

LOVED THE BOOK? LET'S HELP OTHERS DISCOVER THE MAGIC TOO!

Dear Herbalist,

By now, you've steeped teas, infused oils, probably made your kitchen smell like a cross between a forest and a spa, and, most importantly, you've started (or deepened) your journey into the world of herbal wisdom. First off, I'm beyond thrilled you chose to walk this path with me. If this book has helped you feel more connected to nature, more empowered in your health, or even just given you a moment of joy as you sipped a homemade chamomile tea, then my heart is full.

Now, I have one tiny request—and trust me, it's quick, painless, and means the world to me: ***Would you mind leaving a review on Amazon?***

You see, in the vast world of books, reviews are like little breadcrumbs of encouragement. They help other curious souls (just like you!) find this book and feel confident taking their first step into the magic of herbalism. Whether it's a short note about your favorite recipe, a thumbs-up for the tea blends, or just a "hey, this was pretty cool," every review counts.

Not only does your feedback help others, but it also helps me, Barbara Nicole, keep growing this community of budding herbalists. Plus, I'd love to know what you think! What did you try first? What surprised you? Did your windowsill herb garden take over your kitchen (it happens to the best of us)?

So here's my shameless pitch: ***If you've enjoyed this book and it's***

sparked a little more green magic in your life, hop over to Amazon and let me know! *If you didn't love it as much as I'd hoped, hey, I still want to hear about it.*

You, my dear reader, are the roots of this herbal community. Your support allows this wisdom to reach more hands, more hearts, and more homes. Together, we're growing something truly beautiful.

Thank you for being part of this journey, for trusting me as your herbal guide, and for spreading the love (and reviews!) to others. I'm raising a big mug of nettle tea to you—cheers to all the healing, growing, and experimenting ahead!

With gratitude,
Barbara Nicole :)

ABOUT ME

I'm Barbara Nicole, and I'm not a professional herbalist—just a passionate learner who fell head over heels for the incredible world of plants. Over the years, I've learned everything I know about herbs through hands-on experience, trial and error (oh, plenty of error!), and a deep curiosity about how nature can support our well-being.

I started small—brewing teas, experimenting with simple remedies, and growing herbs on my windowsill. Slowly, what began as a hobby turned into a way of life. I've built a home apothecary that I adore, and I've seen firsthand how empowering it is to make your own remedies. That's why I wrote this book: to share what I've learned with you.

You don't need to be an expert to start—just a willingness to learn, a respect for nature, and a little courage to try something new. I believe herbalism is for everyone, and my hope is that this book will inspire you to start your own journey, one tea, tincture, or salve at a time.

Thank you for letting me share this part of my life with you. I'm so excited to see how the wisdom of herbs transforms your home and your heart, just as it did mine.

Made in the USA
Las Vegas, NV
02 January 2025